Medically Unexplained Symptoms

Robert W. Baloh

Medically Unexplained Symptoms

A Brain-Centered Approach

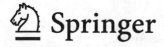 Springer

Robert W. Baloh
Department of Neurology
University of California
Los Angeles, CA
USA

ISBN 978-3-030-59180-9   ISBN 978-3-030-59181-6   (eBook)
https://doi.org/10.1007/978-3-030-59181-6

This Copernicus imprint is published by the registered company Springer Nature Switzerland AG
The registered company address is: Gewerbestrasse 11, 6330 Cham, Switzerland

"The greatest discovery of my generation is that a human being can alter his life by altering his attitudes."

William James

Foreword

Over the ages, doctors have always struggled with patients whose symptoms have no clear medical explanation. Such patients challenge the most essential tenets of medicine. This is not a phenomenon buried in the distant past. All evidence suggests that patients with medically unexplained complaints are as frequent as ever, and maybe even more frequent. The only difference is that the disorders are given different names. As science advances, the cryptic disorders mutate and adapt to the new environment. They are memes that copy themselves with high fidelity and spread across the world, now very rapidly, facilitated by mass media. This is a major problem that causes untold disability and misery. Understanding the problem requires a deep knowledge of the history of medicine and the efforts that have been expended to understand and treat these disorders.

Dr. Robert W. Baloh, a distinguished neurologist with special expertise in vestibular neurology, has had a long career helping patients with dizziness, one of the most prevalent of the symptoms that often lead to no definite diagnosis. From this starting point, he has studied the history of medically unexplained symptoms and articulated a unifying hypothesis, linking them together in a compelling and neuroscientifically explicable continuum.

After beginning with an overview of common medically unexplained symptoms, Dr. Baloh reviews the history of the concept of hysteria in ancient times, followed by the nineteenth century, which many called the golden age of hysteria, through the twentieth century and into present time. His descriptions of the eminent figures in this story are vivid and humane. The reader can really be transported into the various eras and empathize with the efforts of the doctors and scientists to understand and treat these illnesses. Descriptions of the followers of Hippocrates, Briquet, Charcot, Mitchell, Freud, Breuer, Cannon, Selye, and Engel are compelling and reflect both the times and the people. One can appreciate Baloh's hypothesis that the nature of the symptoms in any given period reflects both the training and biases of the physician-scientists and the events of the time. Thus, major societal stressors, such as war and disease, are reflected in the nature of the unexplained symptoms, amplified by the reporting of the events by the media, which, by its very nature, exaggerates the gravity of the episodes.

Baloh then describes the various biological and psychological mechanisms that explain psychosomatic symptoms. The descriptions of the theories are sophisticated and scientifically accurate but are written in such a way that they are understandable to a professional or lay reader who has a genuine interest in these fascinating conditions and their societal consequences. Next, Baloh devotes three chapters to the most common psychosomatic symptoms: pain in the back, abdomen, and head; fibromyalgia/chronic fatigue syndrome; and chronic dizziness. The book ends with a look into the future, including modern techniques such as deep brain stimulation and transcranial magnetic stimulation.

The unifying hypothesis that all of these protean syndromes are manifestations of the brain's response to stress comes through loud and clear. This approach is sympathetic to patients, in that it explicitly states that these experiences are "real" and not imaginary or malingering and that they are all explicable based on a deep understanding of how the brain has evolved in the face of various environmental threats. Many have predicted in various eras that hysteria is dead, but, indeed, it is alive and well in the modern world.

Martin A. Samuels, MD, MACP, FRCP, FANA, FAAN, DSc(Hon)
Miriam Sydney Joseph Distinguished Professor of Neurology
Harvard Medical School
Boston, MA, USA
Founding Chair, Emeritus
Department of Neurology
Brigham and Women's Hospital
Boston, MA, USA

Preface

"Man is more sick, uncertain, changeable, indeterminate than any other animal . . . he is *the sick animal*"

Friedrich Nietzsche [1]

On a daily basis, we are bombarded with sensational stories in the mass media about the advances in modern-day medical science. People with "incurable" cancer are being cured, people with heart disease and stroke have their lives saved as blocked arteries are opened, and people with genetic diseases are identified and treated before they become sick. We are led to believe that modern medicine has all the answers. Yet, for the majority of people who visit a doctor, no identifiable cause is found for their symptoms, so-called medically unexplained symptoms, or MUS for short [2]. Making matters worse, many of these people have the most common symptoms of all – chronic pain, fatigue, and dizziness. As a rule, doctors don't do much for these symptoms; they may even make the symptoms worse.

Although one might reasonably assume that it is abnormal to have symptoms, population studies suggest just the opposite – it is actually more normal to have symptoms than not to have symptoms. A 2014 national telephone survey of New Zealand residents found that the median number of symptoms experienced in the prior week was five and about a quarter of the people had ten or more symptoms [3]. Only 10% of people reported that they had no symptoms in the prior week. The top three reported symptoms were back pain (38%), fatigue (36%), and headache (35%). There is little doubt that current-day people complain of symptoms more than people did in the past [4]. Modern-day people believe that they are sick on a regular basis. When Americans were randomly surveyed as to how many bouts of illness they had over the past few months, those polled in the late 1920s reported 82 episodes of illness from all causes per 100 people, whereas those polled in 1981 reported 212 episodes per 100 people, a 158% increase [5]. This increase in perceived illness is remarkable considering the advances in medical science that occurred in the twentieth century. Since it is unlikely that people in the early twentieth century have fewer symptoms than people in the late twentieth century, modern-day people are more likely to interpret their symptoms as illness compared to those in the past.

Many people, the so-called "worried well," constantly worry about having a serious illness. They are preoccupied with bodily symptoms, amplifying and misinterpreting any bodily symptom that they perceive. With widespread availability of the internet, the first step is usually to Google the symptom and find a long list of disease candidates. People tend to attribute their symptoms to a disease, such as a woman with headaches who is sure she has a brain tumor or a man with dizziness who is sure he is having a stroke. What people think they have is important in the development of illness, since these beliefs are particularly susceptible to "shaping" or "reframing" by health professionals and the mass media. For example, a person who has experienced vague gastrointestinal symptoms for years reads an article about colitis in the Los Angeles Times and becomes convinced that the symptoms are due to that disease. With the recent COVID-19 pandemic, numerous patients with chronic coughs, body aches, and fatigue presented to emergency rooms around the world sure that they had the virus only to test negative. The result of increased somatic awareness is that more people define themselves as patients and more seek help from healthcare professionals than in the past.

But why can't doctors identify the cause of these common symptoms? After all, we have a wide range of highly sensitive diagnostic tests. MRI can identify minute damage in any organ, including the brain. Therein lies the rub. Most people with MUS do not have damage to any body organ. Their symptoms are psychosomatic, caused by physiological changes (changes in chemistry and connectivity) in the brain that are not seen on MRI or identified with any current laboratory test. As we will see throughout this book, the cause of psychosomatic symptoms is a complex interaction between nature and nurture, between biological and psychosocial factors. Slight variations in genes that code for key proteins in the brain can predispose to developing symptoms. A wide variety of biological agents, external and internal, can alter brain function either during development or at the time of onset of symptoms. Psychosocial factors play an important role in initiating and propagating the symptoms. A person's beliefs and expectations, informed by medical professionals and the mass media, can alter and mold the pattern of the symptoms. Psychosomatic symptoms are as real and as severe as the symptoms associated with structural damage. In most cases, the same brain pathways are activated, regardless of whether the symptom is due to structural damage or not, and both types of symptoms have the exact same effect on the person suffering from them. They can be incapacitating and life altering.

Part of the problem is that doctors are not trained to deal with common, everyday symptoms. In modern-day medicine, doctors are trained to rely on laboratory tests to determine whether or not someone is sick. This strategy can lead to the bizarre situation in which people who feel well but have abnormal laboratory tests are told they are sick, whereas people who are sick but have normal laboratory tests are told they are well and the sickness is all in their head. Patient demands and medical-legal risks are reasons doctors give for ordering large numbers of laboratory tests, including MRI of the brain. People expect the most advanced testing available. They are no longer willing to accept reassurance based on experience. However, the process of ordering sophisticated tests and finding nonspecific incidental abnormalities can reinforce the patient's fear of a serious underlying medical problem.

Confidence in doctors has gradually eroded from the early twentieth century to the early twenty-first century. The veneration of doctors common in the past has been replaced by suspicion and mistrust in many cases. People with MUS, in particular, express their frustration with physicians, often shopping from doctor to doctor but never happy with the diagnosis they receive from any of them. Psychosocial factors are behind most patients with MUS, but doctors are understandably reluctant to make a diagnosis of psychosomatic illness. Most have seen patients initially told their symptoms were psychogenic only to be later found to have a biological disease. In our current medical system, physician time is a highly limited commodity, and most physicians don't feel they have the time to listen to the complicated symptom history reported by patients with MUS. Furthermore, discussing and explaining psychosocial implications with patients is very time-consuming and may initially be met with skepticism and even outright hostility.

What is the role of psychiatrists in dealing with MUS? Unfortunately, psychiatrists currently have a very limited role. Patients with MUS usually have little use for psychiatrists and their "talk therapy," and even the suggestion of a referral to a psychiatrist can trigger a hostile reaction from the patient. At the same time, psychiatrists have traditionally had a difficult time dealing with somatic symptoms like pain, fatigue, and dizziness. Since the twentieth century, psychiatric training has moved away from the body and focused on the mind, so that most psychiatrists are ill-prepared to deal with somatic complaints. As we will see, patients with MUS are often bounced back and forth between psychiatrists and other medical specialists who refuse to accept responsibility for the symptoms.

In this book, I address the difficult problem of managing patients with MUS in our modern-day society from both historical and contemporary perspectives. I provide historical background for all concepts, because it is impossible to understand current concepts without knowing the historical context. After an initial overview chapter, Chaps. 2, 3, and 4 focus on the history of psychosomatic illness starting with the ancient concept of hysteria and its evolution through neurasthenia and neurosis to modern-day psychosomatic illness. Chapters 5 and 6 cover the basic mechanisms for psychosomatic symptoms, biological and psychosocial. I have attempted to provide explanatory background material as much as possible in Chap. 5, but the neuroscience "jargon" may prove daunting to some lay readers. Chapter 5 could easily be skipped and used as a reference source without affecting the overall message. Chapters 7, 8, and 9 address the most common MUS, chronic pain (lower back, abdomen, and head), fatigue, and dizziness, and Chap. 10 provides an overview of treatment for psychosomatic symptoms. Each chapter ends with a brief overview paragraph. I provide a brain-centered approach for understanding the cause and treatment of symptoms. If people are to accept psychosocial factors as a cause of MUS, they must understand that there are underlying brain mechanisms to explain the symptoms. Although there are unsolved questions regarding some of these mechanisms, psychosomatic illnesses are just like any other neurological illnesses; they are due to changes in brain function.

Los Angeles, CA, USA   Robert W. Baloh

References

1. Nietzsche F. On the genealogy of morals and Ecce Homo. Translated by W. Kaufmann and R. J. Hollingdale. New York: Random; 1967. Quoted in Morris D. Illness and Culture in the Postmodern Age. Berkeley, CA: University of California Press; 1998.
2. O'Leary D. Why bioethics should be concerned with medically unexplained symptoms. Am J Bioethics 2018;18:6–15.
3. Petrie KJ, Faasse K, Crichton F, Grey A. How common are symptoms? Evidence from a New Zealand national telephone survey. BMJ Open 2014;4:e005374.
4. Stewart DE. The changing faces of somatization. Psychosomatics 1990;31:153–8.
5. Shorter E. From paralysis to fatigue: a history of psychosomatic illness in the modern era. New York: Free Press; 1992. p. 296.

Contents

Overview of Medically Unexplained Symptoms

1

All illness—not just that relegated to the limbo of the psychosomatic—is to some extent constructed by the belief systems of patients, the expectations of practitioners, and the surrounding cultural milieu.

Neil Scheurich [1].

Medically unexplained symptoms (MUS) are symptoms that remain a mystery despite extensive medical evaluation. Even after long-term follow up, the cause remains unidentified in the great majority of cases. Although there is broad agreement that most of these people have psychosomatic symptoms, they are often given a medical diagnosis and receive medical treatments, a process called medicalization [2]. Physicians don't cause the symptoms, but by suggesting that the symptoms may be the harbinger of a potentially serious disease they can increase the symptoms. Furthermore, providing the patient with test results of questionable significance can also amplify the problem. A classic vicious cycle develops whereby the patient focuses on the symptoms and the heightened scrutiny further magnifies the symptoms. There is a strong trend toward increasing somatization and medicalization in modern-day societies.

One theme that will become obvious as this book unfolds is that people are generally uncomfortable with a diagnosis of psychosomatic illness. Many reject it outright with reactions like: "Are you saying this is all in my head?" or "I don't have a psychiatric problem." As I began to write about psychosomatic illness, it became apparent that the meaning of psychogenic is opaque and that there still is no agreed-upon definition. In basic use, it means an illness with a psychological cause rather than an organic cause. But what does that mean? Symptoms due to psychogenic and organic causes are identical to the person experiencing the symptoms. Furthermore, psychosocial factors are important for *all* neurological diseases, including those due to brain tumors, multiple sclerosis and Parkinson disease. The same brain pathways are activated regardless of the underlying mechanism for the symptoms, organic, psychogenic or some combination of the two. They are all neurological symptoms.

R. W. Baloh, *Medically Unexplained Symptoms*,
https://doi.org/10.1007/978-3-030-59181-6_1

The prefix "psycho" has Greek roots in the word *psyche,* meaning spirit or soul. Since the concept of a supernatural soul separate from the physical body has largely been relegated to religious belief, with modern use, the psyche is the mind, the parts of the brain that allow a person to perceive, think rationally and have conscious awareness of being a unique entity. Although most scientists would agree that the mind is in the brain, exactly where and how it is in the brain is much less clear. Modern neuroscience is making some inroads into understanding how the mind is organized, but there is still a long way to go. A critical component of brain function is the ability to learn, and the brain is uniquely designed to learn new information by making associations. People rapidly learn a wide range of behaviors, good and bad, just as they learn history and geography. Many of these behaviors are molded by the society and culture in which they live. With learning, physical changes occur in the chemistry and connections in the brain that can be long-lasting and even permanent (called neuroplasticity). But despite the brain's remarkable learning capabilities, it has flaws and limitations. The brain can be fooled based on prior expectations and beliefs and is highly susceptible to suggestion. Psychosomatic illness is a learned behavior, and the changes that occur in the brain with psychosomatic illness are as real as those that occur in the brain with organic illness.

Pain and Fibromyalgia

Joanne Germanotta is a superstar who by age 30 achieved more acclaim than most entertainers achieve in a lifetime. Her energy level on stage seems boundless; she performs unbelievable body contortions and balancing acts, yet she can be incapacitated for days, writhing in pain, too fatigued to get out of bed. Germanotta was diagnosed with fibromyalgia, a mysterious disease characterized by generalized pain and fatigue along with many other debilitating symptoms for which there is no known cure. Despite having a cadre of therapists at her disposal, she had to cancel a major European musical tour because of her illness. Germanotta, better known as "Lady Gaga," provided insight into her struggles with fame and fibromyalgia in a documentary airing on Netflix, *Gaga: Five Foot Two* [3]. In the documentary she provides a glimpse into her personal struggles, the stress of constantly being in the spotlight and living with chronic pain. This documentary has been an inspiration to patients suffering from this debilitating disorder and also provides insight into the complex interaction between the mind and body with chronic illness [4].

Most physicians agree that there are major psychosocial factors involved in the cause of fibromyalgia. As with all illnesses, however, biological factors are also important, including genetic susceptibility variants, earlier life experiences with illness and pain and hormonal changes associated with stress. Since the pain with fibromyalgia is as severe as any organic cause of pain, one might reasonably ask: Is there a difference between psychogenic and organic pain? Based on current understanding of brain pain mechanisms, the answer is no, there is no clear boundary between "organic" and "psychogenic" pain. With chronic pain, regardless of the cause, chemical and structural changes occur in brain pain pathways, producing "central sensitization" (see Chap. 5). Complicating matters further, organic factors such as infection and injury can initiate pain, and psychosocial factors such as fear and stress can determine whether it resolves or becomes chronic.

The pioneering American neurologist, S. Weir Mitchell, spent much of his career studying pain, both organic and psychogenic in origin, and recognized that psychogenic pain could be as bad as the most severe pain experienced by soldiers injured during the American Civil War. In his monograph, *Lectures on Diseases of the Nervous System, Especially in Women,* published in 1881, he described a 19-year-old woman who came to him on a stretcher with her eyes covered to protect them from sunlight, unable to walk because of constant severe pain throughout her body. He diagnosed her with neurasthenia, a common psychogenic diagnosis at the time, and after treating her with his famous rest cure, during which she was confined to bed and fed large amounts of high-calorie food for several weeks, she gradually improved (see Chap. 3 for more details). After returning home she wrote a letter to Mitchell indicating that her pain began with mental and social strain. "I had for two years before that time suffered from a weak back, had felt constantly tired, spent much of my time on the bed, taken but little exercise…One thing I want to say in extenuation of myself, and that is that the pain was real, not fancied. Whatever its cause or however easily it might have been averted, it was genuine suffering at the time…" [5]. Although many of his contemporary physicians were less understanding, Mitchell was well aware that psychogenic pain was as real as any other type of pain.

Even observing another person suffering from pain can activate parts of the brain involved in emotion, the limbic system, and produce pain in the observer [6]. In 1892, the French physician Paul Joire described a young man who after watching his sister suffer excruciating abdominal pain while passing a bile duct stone (biliary colic) developed similar pain himself. "His acts and his complaints were absolutely identical to those of his sister: he emitted the same cries, he grasped at the right side with the same clasping fingers, as if to tear out what was hurting him. After a certain time, this same pain seemed to radiate towards the epigastric region, the chest and the lower abdomen. He writhed upon the bed 8 days later in exactly the same manner as his sister. The scene could not be more perfectly imitated, and one might indeed have believed in a true hepatic colic, had the end of the attack not furnished evidence of a quite different origin" [7]. The young man went into a typical hysterical fit, and the pain disappeared.

Although pain has been a recognized part of hysteria by the ancient Greeks, it wasn't until the nineteenth century that physicians began to focus on the nature of hysterical pain. In the 1830s the English physician John Conolly emphasized the variety and severity of different pains suffered by patients with hysteria. He noted that the pain could be very intense, like a nail being driven into the forehead, "clavus hystericus," or excruciating abdominal pain mimicking inflammation of the peritoneum [8]. In his groundbreaking 1846 book on hysteria, French physician Hector Landouzy wrote: "One of the invariant characteristics of hysterical pain is its prodigious intensity, in the absence of local findings capable of explaining the violence of the distress. One gets a sense of this in the shrieks that the patients emit when the affected part is touched in the slightest. I remember two hysterics who, in hopes of disencumbering themselves of pain, asked in the one case for a knee amputation, in the other…resection of the sciatic nerve and the extraction of the head of the femur [thigh bone]" [9].

Although generalized body pain has been part of psychogenic illnesses such as hysteria and neurasthenia since ancient times, in modern times the symptom has become the foundation of a separate syndrome: fibromyalgia. Modern patients are less willing to accept a psychogenic explanation for their symptoms, and they want validation of their symptoms by having them attributed to an organic cause [10]. Physicians play a critical role in shaping and propagating patient symptoms and defining illnesses, and like patients, most physicians are uncomfortable with a psychosomatic diagnosis and prefer to lump clinical symptoms into a specific disease category with an organic cause. Many feel uncomfortable even raising the topic of a psychosomatic illness. The modern-day practice of medicine frequently consists of forming a long list of organic diseases and ordering tests to rule them in or out. This approach doesn't work well with psychosomatic illness. It typically worsens the symptoms, like throwing fuel on the fire.

Brain Flaws

Although the human brain is a remarkable organ with a wide range of unique capabilities, it has "design flaws" that make it vulnerable to suggestion and manipulation. Advertisers and politicians routinely take advantage of these flaws to influence our behavior with regard to purchases and voting. The design flaws can be traced to both nature and nurture. The brain evolved over millions of years from about 300 nerve cells in the round worm, to about 20,000 nerve cells in the sea snail (discussed in Chap. 5), to about 90 billion nerve cells in modern humans. The process of evolution is not neat and ordered but rather haphazard with complex interactions between primitive modules deep in the brain and more recently evolved modules in the cerebral cortex. Many of our emotions and behaviors are ingrained in the primitive deep brain modules encoded in our genes. For example, fear, the most basic of all emotions, plays a prominent role in all of our lives, and yet it is only partially under our conscious control. In evolutionary terms, fear plays an important protective role in saving animals from life-threatening dangers such as poisons and predators, the "flight or fight" response. If a species is to reproduce it must stay alive. But an evolutionary trait, hard-wired in our genes, that was helpful for our distant ancestors can be a design flaw in in the brain of modern humans.

In his book, *Brain Bugs: How the Brain's Flaws Shape Our Lives*, UCLA neuroscientist, Dean Buonomano identified two important causes for the power of fear over reasoning: "First the genetic subroutines that determine what we are hardwired to fear were not only written for a different time and place, but also much of the code was written for a different species altogether. Our archaic neural operating system never received the message that predators and strangers are no longer as dangerous as they once were, and that there are more important things to fear…The second cause for our fear related brain bugs is that we are too well prepared to learn fear through observation. Observational learning evolved before the emergence of language, writing, TV and Hollywood – before we were able to learn about things that happened in the real world. Because vicarious learning is in part unconsciousness, it seems to be partially resistant to reason and ill-prepared to distinguish fact from fiction" [11]. No wonder many Americans fear being injured or killed by a terrorist attack much more than they fear being injured or killed in an automobile accident, even though the latter is many-fold more likely to occur than the former. These design flaws in our brain's software make us susceptible to irrational fears that can change the chemistry and physiology of our brain and body and produce a wide range of symptoms. This type of narrative using an analogy with computer software problems was shown to be useful for explaining their symptoms to patients with fibromyalgia [12].

Fear

The amygdala is an evolutionary primitive structure, part of the limbic system deep in the brain, which is critical for the expression and learning of fear and developing anxiety (see Chap. 5). Damage to the amygdala results in fearless, emotionally flat animals. Sudden unexpected odors or sounds triggered fear and the "flight or fight" response in our primitive ancestors as they wandered through the forest. Just as Pavlov's dogs learned to associate ringing of a bell with increased salivation, repeated threatening sounds led to increased activation of the amygdala fear-anxiety pathways over time. Fear and associated anxiety are part of most psychogenic illnesses. For example, phobias are manifested by exaggerated, inappropriate fear of a specific circumstance, such as being confined in an enclosed space or driving on a Los Angeles freeway. With post-traumatic stress disorder (PTSD), fear and anxiety become pervasive, triggered by thoughts or events that remind the sufferer of a prior traumatic experience, for example, slamming of a door reminding a soldier of a battle experience. The fear circuits of the brain have become conditioned to respond excessively to these usually benign circumstances. But why does fear have so much power over our reasoning ability? The amygdala is closely interrelated with the prefrontal cortex, the evolutionary new brain area critical for "executive functions" such as decision making and keeping primitive emotions under control. These brain modules are constantly working on a compromise between emotions and reason. But the number of nerve connections from the amygdala to the prefrontal cortex outnumbers the connections from the prefrontal cortex to the amygdala [13]. Thus, there may be an anatomical substrate for emotions to dominate executive functions such as rational thinking (see Chap. 5). Could it be possible to increase the connectivity from the prefrontal cortex to the amygdala and thus better control primitive emotions like fear? Cognitive behavioral therapy and magnetic or electrical stimulation of the prefrontal cortex may in fact do this, and modern-day brain imaging techniques can be used to document the change (these topics will be discussed in more detail in Chap. 10).

Anxiety

Like pain, anxiety has been part of psychosomatic illness since ancient times, but the concept that anxiety may be biological became popular with Walter Cannon's "fight or flight" hypothesis in the 1920s (see Chap. 5). Cannon produced many of the features of anxiety by triggering the release of adrenaline from the adrenal gland or by injecting adrenaline into an animal. With improved understanding of the limbic system and its connections to the hypothalamus and key brainstem centers, a neurobiological model for anxiety evolved. As noted earlier, the amygdala is a key structure for generating the fear response and cortical control of the amygdala is critical for modulating the response. Impaired cortical control of the amygdala can result in misinterpretation of body cues and an inappropriate activation of the fear network. Slight variants in the genes that code for key proteins in the fear network help explain why certain people are more sensitive to developing anxiety attacks [14]. Variations in the genes that code for proteins associated with the neurotransmitter serotonin have received the greatest attention because drugs that elevate the level of serotonin in the brain are useful for treating anxiety.

As with chronic pain, anxiety is associated with "central sensitization." Patients with anxiety are hypersensitive to sensory stimuli, including light, sound, motion, pain, and smell. They often startle with just the slightest touch. The paradox is that despite the heightened sensitivity, overall brain function is inefficient. When discussing this problem with patients, I often use the analogy of a motor running out of gear. Patients have difficulty concentrating and focusing their attention (so-called brain fog). They are easily distracted and are less productive in their work. They have difficulty getting to sleep and never feel rested. Anxiety occurs with most psychosomatic symptoms, and it is part of many degenerative neurological conditions and may even be the initial manifestation of a neurological disease.

Patients with anxiety frequently present to physicians with somatic symptoms such as pain, fatigue and dizziness, even though they are aware that they also feel anxious. Often, they conclude that the symptoms are causing their anxiety. For example, a middle-age woman complained of what she called "brain fog" dating back more than 10 years [15]. She had seen 57 different physicians for the problem and provided a large bundle of carefully annotated records to prove it. The brain fog was constant and was associated with difficulty concentrating and difficulty sleeping. In the past she had been diagnosed with fibromyalgia and suffered from daily pain throughout her body. She also complained of difficulty with memory and would forget names and where she had placed objects. Her symptoms became much worse when one of the physicians she consulted suggested that she might have a rare type of dementia. Over the 10 years she had undergone seven MRI examinations of the brain, all of which were normal, and her neurological examination was completely normal. She spent her days mostly sitting in a chair at home since she was convinced that her symptoms were worse with any type of physical activity or by being in a noisy or crowded area. Doctors told her to avoid activities that aggravated her brain fog.

What does this tragic story tell us about psychosomatic symptoms and how they are being managed in the United States? The fact that she saw 57 different physicians for her problem may seem extreme, but it is by no means a record. Why do patients see the need to visit so many different physicians? They typically have symptoms in many subspecialty areas, so they seek out subspecialty physicians for each symptom. Primary care physicians who might be able to see the overall picture have limited time to address the complicated symptom list, and many don't feel competent dealing with symptoms such as pain and dizziness. But as noted earlier, the process of ordering tests and suggesting serious organic diseases can be counterproductive and ultimately lead to worsening of symptoms. What is needed is someone (preferable with grey hair and exuding confidence) who can reassure the patient that the symptoms are real and not just in their head and that they are caused by changes in the brain that can be reversed with treatment. A referral to a psychiatrist for cognitive behavioral therapy and possibly pharmacological therapy might be part of the treatment process, but, as noted in the Preface, many psychiatrists are very uncomfortable with somatic symptoms such as pain, fatigue and dizziness. They themselves may initiate the "doctor chase" by raising the possibility of organic illnesses and sending the patient to multiple medical subspecialists.

Stress

Everyone has experienced stress, yet most of us would have a difficult time saying exactly what stress represents. Psychologists have defined emotional stress as a process whereby environmental demands exceed a person's ability to cope. The feeling of being unable to cope and how we react to that feeling can affect our overall health and our susceptibility to illness. Short periods of emotional stress may be no problem and may even improve performance in an athlete or a scholar. But longer periods of emotional stress are nearly always harmful, causing emotional and physical problems. At work, stress can cause conflicts with colleagues, poor concentration, and performance anxiety along with subpar performance; at home, stress can lead to family discord, fatigue, insomnia, overeating and overuse of alcohol. The negative health effects of chronic stress are alarming. Up to 75% of patient visits to doctors in the United States are in some way related to chronic stress [16]. This includes a wide variety of physical complaints, including headache, abdominal pain, low back pain, chronic fatigue, sleep disorders, dizziness and depression. An estimated 80% to 90% of work-related accidents are due to stressful personal problems and the worker's inability to handle stress, and about half of lost workdays are stress-related.

But is it stress or the perception of stress that causes the problem? Studies in people who complain of frequent symptoms (often called somatic awareness or somatic focus) tend to have an overall negative affect, meaning that they feel a high level of stress and dissatisfaction even when there is little environmental stress [17]. The number of reported daily symptoms is much better correlated with negative affect than with objective measures of health status. It follows that symptom questionnaires commonly used by health professionals to screen patients are a better measure of negative affect than of health status and that perceived stress is as deadly as real stress.

One of the most studied manifestations of stress is its effect on the immune system [18]. The notion that there is a connection between one's physical health and the brain and emotions dates back to ancient times. More recently, the field of psychoneuroimmunology has focused on the interaction of the mind/brain on the body's defense against infection and cancer. There is no doubt that stress suppresses the immune system and makes one more vulnerable to infections, particularly viral infections such as the common cold [19]. Small messenger molecules called cytokines that are released by a variety of immune cells during stress can initiate an inflammatory response and stress-related sickness. Injecting cytokines into animals can produce a systemic illness with severe generalized fatigue. Drugs that block cytokines can improve chronic fatigue in patients with rheumatoid arthritis [20]. Organic and psychogenic suppression of the immune system seem to work through the same mechanisms (discussed in Chap. 5).

Chronic Fatigue Syndrome

Chronic fatigue syndrome is associated with fibromyalgia and manifested by severe persistent fatigue and a variety of other symptoms, including dizziness, pain and cognitive impairment. Many consider it part of a disease spectrum: the fibromyalgia/chronic fatigue syndrome. One of the best lay descriptions of chronic fatigue syndrome was provided by the writer Laura Hillenbrand, in an article published in 2003 in the *New Yorker* entitled "A Sudden Illness, How My Life Changed" [21]. "One morning, I woke to find my limbs leaden. I tried to sit up but couldn't. I lay in bed, listening to my apartment-mates move through their morning routines. It was two hours before I could stand. On the walk to the bathroom, I had to drag my shoulder along the wall to stay upright." This occurred during her third year of college and she had to drop out of college and return home where she spent the next 3 years barely able to move about. She finally improved but had a relapse after a terrifying experience when she was trapped in an automobile during a violent rainstorm. "For as long as two months at a time, I couldn't get down the stairs. Bathing became nearly impossible. Once a week or so, I sat on the edge of the tub and rubbed a washcloth over myself. The smallest exertion plunged me into a 'crash'. First, my legs would weaken and I'd lose the strength to stand. Then I wouldn't be able to sit up. My arms would go next, and I'd be unable to lift them. I couldn't roll over. Soon, I would lose the strength to speak. Only my eyes were capable of movement. At the bottom of each breath, I would wonder if I'd be able to draw the next one." Along with the extreme fatigue she had many other symptoms, including sore throat, nausea, dizziness, chills, sweating and confusion. "In conversation, I'd think of one word but say something completely unrelated: "hotel" became "plankton"; "cup" came out "elastic." I couldn't hang on to a thought long enough to carry it through a sentence. When I tried to cross the street, the motion of the cars became so disorienting that I couldn't move. I was at a sensory distance from the world, as if I were wrapped in clear plastic."

Hillenbrand's experience with physicians typifies the medical profession's schizophrenic approach in dealing with this strange illness. First the doctors thought she had an infection, probably strep throat, but she did not respond to penicillin or any other antibiotics. She saw a specialist in internal medicine, and after extensive testing he told her the problem was not in her body but in her mind and that she should see a psychiatrist. The psychiatrist told her he would bet his reputation that she was mentally healthy and suffering from a physical illness. The internist's response to the psychiatrist's report was "find another psychiatrist." Neurologists ran tests but could find no explanation for her symptoms. Several doctors thought it was a virus, possibly mono, and when she was referred to a "mono doctor" he told her that she had a positive blood antibody test for Epstein-Barr virus (discussed in Chap. 8). He confidently made the diagnosis of "Epstein-Barr viral syndrome" and began her on a nutritional-supplement pill that he touted "cured" the condition. But after multiple visits she became disillusioned not only because of the lack of improvement but because she found out that the doctor had diagnosed everyone working in his office and also her mother who accompanied her as having Epstein-Barr viral syndrome. After seeing a woman doctor several times, the doctor told her, "I don't know why you keep coming here." The doctor then went into the waiting room and told her mother, "When is she going to realize that her problems are all in her head?" Before completely giving up on doctors, she decided to follow the suggestion of the psychiatrist and visit Dr. John G. Bartlett, the chief of the Division of Infectious Diseases at Johns Hopkins University School of Medicine. After reviewing her records and performing numerous tests, Dr. Bartlett told her she had a "real" disease, chronic fatigue syndrome. The cause was unknown, but he suspected a virus, although Epstein-Barr virus was definitely not the cause. He could offer no treatment but suggested that some patients spontaneously recover. When she asked if that meant some don't recover, his response was yes. As strange as it may seem, this consultation seemed to provide some comfort to her, knowing that someone recognized her condition and that the symptoms were "real." But the symptoms continued, and it became a matter of how to live with them.

Dizziness, which took on several forms from "brain fog" to near faint dizziness to frank vertigo, was a prominent feature of her chronic illness. She described how the room began to whirl violently while she was sitting in bed reading a magazine. "I dropped the magazine and grabbed on to the dresser. I felt as though I were rolling and lurching, a ship on the high seas. I clung to the dresser and waited for the feeling to pass, but it didn't… The vertigo wouldn't stop. I didn't lie on my bed so much as ride it as it swung and spun… The furniture flexed and skidded around the room, and the walls folded and unfolded. Every few days there was a sudden plunging sensation, and I would throw my arms out to catch myself… Sleep brought no respite; every dream took place on the deck of a tossing ship, a runaway rollercoaster, a plane caught in violent turbulence, a falling elevator. Looking at anything close-up left me reeling. I couldn't read or write. I rented audiobooks, but I couldn't follow the narratives."

Gradually over time her symptoms improved but she never returned to normal, and there was always the threat of an exacerbation. "One mistake could land me in bed for weeks, so the potential cost of even the most trivial activities, from showering to walking to the mailbox, had to be painstakingly considered. Sometimes I relapsed for no reason at all. Living in perpetual fear of collapse was stressful, but on my good days I was functioning much better." During these good days, she was able to write her best-selling books, *Seabiscuit: An American Legend* (2001) and *Unbroken: A World War II Story of Survival, Resilience, and Redemption* (2010), which combined sold over 13 million copies. The writing was a struggle, as she described, "If I looked down at my work, the room spun, so I perched my laptop on a stack of books in my office... When I was too tired to sit at my desk, I set the laptop up on my bed. When I was too dizzy to read, I lay down and wrote with my eyes closed. Living in my subjects' bodies, I forgot about my own."

How can psychosomatic symptoms be so disabling and so persistent? This woman had a life-long illness that in many ways is worse than some of the most severe organic illnesses such as diabetes and cancer. Yet doctors were baffled and could find no explanation for her symptoms. Serendipitously, while I was reading about Laura Hillenbrand's illness, I received an e-mail asking me to participate in a survey about chronic fatigue syndrome. The first question was: Do you believe that chronic fatigue syndrome is a neurological disease? This question epitomizes the problem that doctors have in dealing with psychosomatic illnesses. Of course, it is a neurological disease and it shouldn't matter what doctors believe. Any neurologist worth his salt who reads Hillenbrand's description of her symptoms will recognize that she has a neurological disease. So it is time to get beyond unproductive conflicts in terminology. Biological and psychosocial factors are important for all neurological diseases. Some diseases may have gross structural changes, whereas others have only physiological changes in the brain, but the end result can be the same, real symptoms.

Diagnostic Uncertainty

Although the great majority of MUS are psychosomatic in origin, MUS and psychosomatic symptoms are not the same thing. Some MUS have biological causes yet to be identified, and others represent benign biological disorders that get better without treatment. Physicians have long known that when the diagnosis is in doubt wait awhile to see if the symptoms go away. With chronic symptoms the big issue is how much biological testing is necessary to rule out a biological cause? There are uncertainties with all medical diagnoses, no matter how many tests are done. In his famous address to medical graduates in the late nineteenth century, the pioneering medical educator William Osler emphasized that physicians must learn to deal with diagnostic uncertainties: "A distressing feature in the life which you are about to enter, a feature which will press hardly upon the finer spirits among you and ruffle their equanimity, is the uncertainty which pertains not only to our science and art, but to the very hopes and fears which makes us men. In seeking absolute truth we aim at the unattainable, and must be content with finding broken portions" [22]. As a rule, doctors don't do a very good job of explaining medical uncertainty to patients particularly with regard to psychosomatic symptoms. Some of the common biological disorders that are misdiagnosed as psychosomatic include autoimmune disorders, rare diseases (genetic and acquired) and numerous disorders in women particularly heart disease. But as suggested earlier, it is much more likely psychosomatic symptoms will be misdiagnosed as biological.

Do psychosomatic illnesses represent a separate category of illness? The prevailing biopsychosocial model of medical practice assumes a spectrum of illnesses from those that are mostly biological to those that are mostly psychosocial but all have some combination of biological and psychosocial factors. As a rule, doctors do a reasonably good job in discussing the biological implications of symptoms but not so good a job in discussing psychosocial implications. To circumvent perceived patient resistance, physicians often use ambiguous and vague terms or avoid the subject altogether. What does the patient expect? When patients present to a physician with what they perceive to be a biological symptom, do they consent for the doctor to assess psychosocial issues? Doctors typically assume such consent since, by tradition dating back to Hippocrates, medical practice mandates that physicians consider the whole person, mind and body. Bioethicist Diane O'Leary, however, pointed out that patients may not necessarily share this conceptual grounding: "In a very basic sense, the patient understands herself to have entered into an implicit contract with the physician where the biological medical care she seeks for her symptoms will be provided for a fee. When the physician ventures into emotional territory instead of offering that biological care, it is not unreasonable to imagine the typical patient might feel this is not what she signed up for—and this presents us with a ready explanation for the resentment patients express in response to psychogenic diagnosis" [23].

Are patients really that resistant to a psychosomatic diagnosis? It is all in the presentation. Clearly, using phrases such as "it's all in your head" or "you need to see a psychiatrist" is doomed to failure. In my experience, most patients are very receptive to discussing psychosocial issues and the effect these issues have on their symptoms. In fact, many complain that their doctors don't take the time to consider these issues. Patients need to have time to tell their stories, and in most instances, they will introduce psychosocial issues themselves if they are given the time. On the other hand, time is a critical element, and in our current medical system, physicians don't feel they have adequate time to address complex psychosocial issues. Ideally, physicians should treat all symptoms alike, querying about possible biological and psychosocial factors so that patients feel their symptoms are being taken seriously. Since psychosocial factors contribute to the cause of all symptoms, physicians should regularly prescribe a variety of treatments such as physical exercise, stress management techniques, coping strategies, good sleep habits and healthy eating for all of their patients. As we will see, such treatments are often the most effective available options, regardless of the cause of the patient's symptoms. Before discussing current thinking on the biological and psychosocial causes of psychosomatic symptoms, it is helpful to look at how these ideas developed historically. This knowledge will provide the necessary background for understanding modern concepts of psychosomatic symptoms.

In Brief

Although the majority of medically unexplained symptoms are psychosomatic in origin, people are often given a medical diagnosis and receive medical treatments for the symptoms. By suggesting that the symptoms may be the harbinger of a potentially serious disease and providing test results of questionable significance, physicians may inadvertently amplify the symptoms. Chronic pain is by far the most common medically unexplained symptom followed by fatigue and dizziness. Stress, defined as an inability to cope, is at the root of most psychosomatic symptoms, and managing stress should be at the center of any treatment program.

References

1. Scheurich N. Hysteria and the medical narrative. Perspect Biol Med. 2000;43:465.
2. Barsky AJ, Borus JF. Somatization and medicalization in the era of managed care. JAMA. 1995;274:1931–4.
3. Netflix documentary, Gaga: Five Foot Two. Director, Chris Moukarbel, Live Nations Productions.
4. Banach JE. Lady Gaga's new Netflix documentary is a rallying cry to those who suffer from chronic pain. Vogue, September 22, 2017.
5. Mitchell SW. Lectures on diseases of the nervous system, especially in women, vol. 1881. London: Royal College of Physicians of Edinburgh. p. 87–8.
6. Osborn J, Derbyshire SWG. Pain sensation evoked by observing injury in others. Pain. 2010;148:268–74.
7. Shorter E. From paralysis to fatigue: a history of psychosomatic illness in the modern era. New York: Free Press; 1992. p. 286.
8. Shorter E. From paralysis to fatigue: a history of psychosomatic illness in the modern era. New York: Free Press; 1992. p. 288.
9. Shorter E. From paralysis to fatigue: a history of psychosomatic illness in the modern era. New York: Free Press; 1992. p. 288.
10. Shorter E. From paralysis to fatigue: a history of psychosomatic illness in the modern era. New York: Free Press; 1992. p. 295.
11. Buonomano D. Brain bugs. How the Brain's flaws shape our lives. New York: WW Norton; 2011. p. 141.
12. Hyland ME, Hinton C, Hill C, Whalley B, Jones RC, Davies AF, et al. Explaining unexplained pain to fibromyalgia patients: finding a narrative that is acceptable to patients and provides a rationale for evidence based interventions. Br J Pain. 2016;10:156–61.
13. Sah P, Westbrook RF, Lüthi A. Fear conditioning and long term potentiation in the amygdala. Ann N Y Acad Sci. 2008;1129:88–95.
14. Bystritsky A, Khalsa SS, Cameron ME, Schiffman J. Current diagnosis and treatment of anxiety disorders. Pharm Ther. 2013;38(1):30–8.
15. Private patient of RWB, details changed to protect privacy.
16. LeDoux JE. The emotional brain. New York: Touchstone; 1996. p. 303.

17. Watson D, Pennebaker JW. Health complaints, stress, and distress: exploring the central role of negative affectivity. Psych Rev. 1989;96:234–54.
18. Segerstrom SC, Miller GE. Psychological stress and the human immune system: a meta-analytic study of 30 years of inquiry. Psychol Bull. 2004;130:601–30.
19. Cohen S, Tyrrell DA, Smith AP. Psychological stress in humans and susceptibility to the common cold. N Engl J Med. 1991;325:606–12.
20. Rider P, Carmi Y, Cohen I. Biologics for targeting inflammatory cytokines, clinical uses, and limitations. Int J Cell Biol 2016, pp1–11.
21. Hillenbrand L. A sudden illness. How my life changed. The New Yorker, 2003 July 7.
22. Osler W. Aequanimatas. With other addresses to medical students, nurses and practitioners of medicine. 3rd ed. Philadelphia: P. Blakiston's Son and Co.; 1932. p. 6–7.
23. O'Leary D. Why bioethics should be concerned with medically unexplained symptoms. Am J Bioeth. 2018;18:8.

Early Ideas on Hysteria

2

> The fundamental point remains: the realm of disease is unstable, with etiologies and nosologies always exhibiting some degree of flux, and doctors are generally no more able than their patients to shake themselves free of the assumptions and prejudices of their era.
>
> Andrew Scull [1].

The term hysteria is derived from the Greek word for the uterus, *hysterika.* In ancient civilizations, it was used to describe a syndrome of nervous irritability, near-faint dizziness (swooning), pain, fatigue, weakness and many other symptoms that were thought to occur uniquely in women. The first clear description of the medical syndrome is found in the *Hippocratic Corpus,* a compilation of writings from the fifth century B.C., many of which are attributed to Hippocrates, the Greek physician considered the father of medicine. Hippocrates and his followers believed that hysteria resulted from a "wandering uterus." As strange as it may seem today, these ancient physicians thought the uterus could physically move throughout body and the type of symptoms experienced depended on where the uterus settled. Exhaustion, lack of water and food, absence of sex and excessive dryness or lightness of the uterus were a few of the many factors that caused it to move. When the uterus moved upward in the woman's body, forcing its way into the crowded places at the center, it could cause the woman to have difficulty breathing, swoon or faint and become speechless. Some ancient physicians likened the uterus to a vicious animal ("an animal within an animal") that erratically moved about and could invade other organs such as the liver, spleen and stomach or prolapse downward into the vagina [2]. Since they thought that it was attracted by fragrant smells and repelled by fetid smells, physicians treated hysteria by rubbing the vagina with honey and having the woman chew cloves of garlic. When the physician diagnosed that the uterus had moved upward in the abdomen, he would manually try to push it back downwards and keep it down by tying a tight bandage below the rib cage.

R. W. Baloh, *Medically Unexplained Symptoms,*
https://doi.org/10.1007/978-3-030-59181-6_2

Hysteria and Female Sexuality

The famous Roman physician, Galen, questioned the wandering uterus theory but believed that the uterus was the seat of the problem, possibly by releasing vapors that moved upward and affected other organs of the body [3]. The cause was sexual deprivation, and the cure was increased sexual activity. Married women with symptoms of hysteria were told to have sex with their husbands, and single women of marriageable age were instructed to marry. For other women (widows, unhappily married and nuns), treatments included vigorous horseback riding, rocking the pelvis on a swing or chair and having a physician or midwife massage the vulva with a finger. This notion that hysteria was a uniquely female disorder that could be treated with sexual activity persisted throughout the Middle Ages and well into modern times. Galen's influence on the routine practice of medicine persisted for well over a thousand years. In the 1600s, Thomas Sydenham, the famous English physician commonly known as the English Hippocrates, noted that only the diagnosis of "fever" was more common than the diagnosis of hysteria in his practice. The famous seventeenth century French surgeon, Ambroise Paré, recommended that patients with hysteria should have more sexual interaction with their husbands. Interestingly, masturbation by the patient was frowned upon and even thought to cause or aggravate the problem. Physicians tried to achieve a "hysterical paroxysm" but did not mention orgasm as the goal of their stimulation treatment. Understanding of female sexual gratification was severely limited at the time, and it was generally felt that the only way for a woman to have "real" sexual gratification was penetration of the vagina by an erect penis and male orgasm.

Most physicians found the process of treating hysteria with their finger tedious and time-consuming, so they turned the task over to midwives [4]. Women of means were referred to spas where they could receive water massage therapy. In America, women were often the owners of these so-called water cure establishments. In the latter half of the nineteenth century, the American physician, George Taylor, built and patented a steam-powered vibrating apparatus to massage the pelvis in women with hysteria. Taylor warned against "overindulgence" with his vibrating apparatus. A few years later, the first battery-powered electromechanical vibrator was developed by the English physician Joseph Mortimer Granville, and although he initially recommended use only for muscle massage, it rapidly became popular for treating hysteria. At the turn of the twentieth century, these devices were marketed for women's health to provide "all the pleasures of youth" and were targeted to men as gifts to put the "pink back in the cheeks" of their wives and girlfriends. A particularly versatile vibrator was advertised in the Sears and Roebuck catalogue that could also be used for a variety of household chores such a churning, grinding and mixing.

Bizarre Behaviors

As suggested earlier, many symptoms have been attributed to hysteria. Nonspecific symptoms such as dizziness, fatigue, weakness, generalized body pain, emotional outbursts, cognitive impairment and headaches were most common. A sensation of suffocating as though one has a ball in the throat restricting breathing was considered characteristic, so-called *globus hystericus*. In the first century A.D. the famous Roman physician Celsus noted that hysterical fits were similar to epileptic fits but usually without the convulsions and the foaming at the mouth. Paralysis, facial and body tics, behaviors such as running, dancing, tumbling and pelvic thrusting, and vocalizations, particularly swearing, were all symptoms exhibited by patients with hysteria.

In the mid-fourteenth century, hundreds of people along the Rhine River valley in Europe developed a strange compulsion to dance [5]. They would dance day and night without pausing to eat or sleep. The behavior migrated to towns throughout Europe and then gradually subsided over a few months. The so-called dancing mania resurfaced more than a century later in Strasbourg, and in this case, it was well documented by physicians and monks in the area. About 400 men, women and children participated, and several dozen died. Around the same time, in the late fifteenth century, an outbreak of bizarre behaviors occurred in nunneries throughout Europe. Groups of nuns would scream and swear, go into a trance-like state and mimic the behavior of dogs or cats or perform lewd behaviors such as lifting up their habits and simulate copulation. Some propositioned priests and claimed to have carnal relations with the devil or Christ.

Not surprisingly, the possibility of possession by demons or the devil was suspected, and many, particularly the nuns, were treated with exorcisms. The possibility of some type of mass poisoning, such as with food contaminated with ergot, was entertained by physicians at the time, but they could find no pattern of food or environmental contamination to explain the phenomena. Most likely these epidemics of bizarre behaviors represented the first documented instances of mass hysteria, now called mass psychogenic illness, defined as the collective occurrence of physical symptoms and related beliefs among two or more persons in the absence of an identifiable pathogen.

Hysteria and the Occult

In the seventeenth century, cases of hysteria attributed to witches' spells provide valuable insight into the disorder and the importance of the environment in which it takes place. Two well-documented instances of witch hysteria occurred in London at the beginning of the century and in Salem, Massachusetts at the end of the century. In 1602, Mary Glover, the 14-year-old daughter of a well-to-do shopkeeper in London, developed a choking sensation while drinking her posset [6]. Her throat seemed to swell so that she could not swallow the creamy liquid. The symptoms began when an elderly neighbor woman, Elizabeth Jackson, came to the house to complain to Mary's mother about her perceived ill treatment by Mary. The symptoms started when Jackson glared and snarled at the young girl. Mary then began having fits of suffocating along with deafness and blindness, typically triggered by trying to eat. They were so severe that the family thought she might die. Mrs. Jackson was heard by other neighbors thanking God for bringing his vengeance on her tormentor. When Mary encountered Mrs. Jackson over the next several days, she would develop bizarre rolling spells, first extending her head backwards like a reverse C and rolling violently backwards and then reversing and bending her head between her legs and rolling forward. It took several women to stop the rolls and keep her from injuring herself.

Over the following weeks Mary developed a variety of other "fits" during which she would writhe and contort her body, prance and dance about the room, and make strange breathing patterns and vocalizations. At times she would shout out praise to God and ask him to deliver her from her afflictions. Mary's bizarre spells were well known throughout London, and devout Puritans and skeptics alike came to witness them. Finally, she was taken to the local Sheriff's office to confront Mrs. Jackson, the accused perpetrator of this evildoing. On this and several subsequent meetings with Mrs. Jackson, Mary would exhibit even more dramatic symptoms with spectacular loud verbal outbursts, wide-eyed trances, tics, and contortions lasting hours. She would forcibly close her mouth and produce a garbled sound through her nostrils that sounded like "hang her." This only occurred in her fits when Mrs. Jackson was present.

Naturally there was skepticism regarding the authenticity of Mary's bizarre behavior. Was she simply trying to get back at Mrs. Jackson, who she perceived as her tormentor? Mary and Mrs. Jackson were ordered to report to Mr. Crooke, the Recorder of London, for further evaluation of the matter. Mr. Crooke first tried to trick Mary by having another woman disguised as Mrs. Jackson come into the room, but Mary did not react. When Mrs. Jackson was disguised and entered the room, Mary immediately went into one of her fits with the strange vocalization through her nose. The Recorder then decided to test Mary during one of her spells during which she would stare but not respond. He brought the flame of a burning candle first to her cheek and then to her eyes as if he were going to burn her, but she did not flinch and remained unblinking. He then placed a ball of burning paper into the palm of her right hand but she showed no reaction, even though she had burns on the hand after she came out of her fit.

A decision was finally made: Mary was bewitched, and the source of her possession was Mrs. Jackson. A trial was held at the Court of Common Pleas with Sir Edmund Anderson, a notorious witch-finding judge, as Chief Justice. At the trial, Edward Jordan, a prominent member of the London College of Physicians, testified that he believed that Elizabeth Jackson was not guilty of witchcraft but rather Mary suffered from a bodily illness, hysteria. He pointed out that it was an affliction of her uterus and subsequently her brain that caused her strange symptoms and that it was to medicine, not the supernatural, that one should look for a cure. But Jordan had to admit that he couldn't prove his diagnosis and that he couldn't guarantee a cure for Mary. Judge Anderson would have none of that and reminded the jury that Mrs. Jackson had stumbled over words in the Lord's Prayer and had the mark of a witch on her body (a wart). The jury convicted Mrs. Jackson of witchcraft, and the judge sentenced her to prison and the pillory. Fortunately for Elizabeth Jackson, her sentence was subsequently suspended because of concerns raised by her supporters, but 2 years later the law was changed to make witchcraft a capital offense, and many women were hanged in London for similar witches' spells.

In 1692 in Salem, Massachusetts, the 9-year-old daughter and 11-year-old niece of a local minister, Samuel Parris, began having strange spells during which they would appear to go into a trance and shout blasphemies and conduct bizarre behaviors such as barking like dogs and dancing, running and tumbling about the room [7]. Word spread about the spells throughout Salem Village, and several additional young girls began to exhibit the same kinds of behaviors. As in the case of Mary Glover, the possibility of evil forces was entertained and when the girls were pressured to explain the source of their spells, they named three women in the village as witches. One was a black slave of the Reverend Paris, Tituba; the second, an unpopular woman who was known to make threats against her neighbors; and the third, a woman who lived with a man for several months before getting married. The town magistrates interviewed the women, and two of them denied being a witch or knowing anything about witches, but Tituba, who had shown a keen interest in the occult, readily confessed and boasted that many other people in Salem were also practicing witchcraft. Over the subsequent months, more than 150 people in Salem were accused of witchcraft, and 14 women and 5 men were sentenced to death by hanging. A 20th victim, farmer Giles Corey, died after being crushed by stones placed on a board that lay on top of him in an effort to gain a confession. The hunt for witches even spread to the nearby village of Andover.

There are several similarities in the illnesses suffered by these young women in seventeenth century London and New England. Wide-eyed staring fits with loss of speech and sight, difficulty swallowing, abnormal breathing with a sensation of suffocating, strange body contortions and writhing, odd postures with motor and vocal tics all were common features. When they occurred in multiple people in the same home or community, the pattern of symptoms tended to be stereotyped. Even in these early times, there was great skepticism about the authenticity of the symptoms. Were these young women malingering, using these bizarre behaviors to gain a social advantage? As with Mary Glover, skeptics, including many physicians, tried to discredit the young women by tricking them to reveal their fakery, but they were remarkably unsuccessful. The young women appeared to be in a trance-like state and were impervious to threat and pain.

Nerves

In the early seventeenth century, little was known about nerves and the brain and their role in controlling behavior. Theories on nerve and brain function were based on mysterious entities such as animal spirits and souls. Rene Decartes, the famous seventeenth century French philosopher, devised an elaborate theory to explain the brain's role in both voluntary and involuntary behavior [8]. He considered nerves to be hollow tubes that were connected with the fluid-filled compartments in the brain called ventricles. For reflex behavior such as withdraw from a painful stimulus, he postulated that thin filaments within each nerve tube controlled tiny valves in the ventricles of the brain that controlled the flow of animal spirits into the nerves. Painful pressure or heat against the skin would move the filaments (like pulling on a rope to ring a bell), open the valves and release animal spirits from the ventricles into the nerve causing a reflex muscle contraction. For voluntary behavior, Decartes proposed that the rational immortal soul, which he localized in the pineal gland, perceived sensations such as pain and pleasure and controlled the flow of spirits by deciding when to open and close the tiny valves within the ventricle. An analogy was a spider sitting at the center of his web aware of any slight movement of a fiber in the web. The soul was separate from the brain and lived on after death. Decartes picked the pineal gland because it was an unpaired structure (since there was only one soul) and was located between the lateral ventricles surrounded by cerebrospinal fluid. Critics immediately pointed out the disturbing facts that the pineal gland was much more prominent in animals lower on the evolutionary scale than in humans and that the pineal gland was located outside of the ventricles and thus not in contact with the spinal fluid.

Decartes theory became very popular, primarily for its simple mechanical explanation of reflex behavior, but there were unintended consequences. It raised an interesting question: Do animals feel pain? A heated debate occurred in the scientific community. Since Catholic religious doctrine, faithfully followed by Decartes, taught that only humans have an immortal soul, it followed that nonhuman animals could not "feel" pain. They had animal spirits in the ventricles of the brain that controlled reflex behavior but lacked an immortal soul to sense the emotion of pain and pleasure (they were automatons). This may seem foolish, because we have all seen animals grimace and moan after injury, suggesting that they are in pain. Decartes dismissed these reactions to injury as automatic reflexes that did not indicate that the animal "feels" pain. The result was that he and his many followers conducted experiments on animals without concern for pain. Not surprisingly, a reactionary antivivisection movement developed.

At the time Descartes published his famous book *Principes de la Philosophie* (Principles of Philosophy) in 1644, Thomas Willis, a young physician in Oxford, England, was busily dissecting hundreds of animals and humans, including many of his own patients who had died from brain diseases. When he examined nerves under a magnifying glass, he noted that they were solid cords, not hollow tubes, so he felt that they must contain very tiny pores for the animal spirits to move through. To Willis animal spirits represented a fundamental force derived from the soul that moved within nerves. He developed methods to remove and preserve the brain from the skull so that he could study it in detail. Willis speculated that the brain itself, not the ventricles, must be the center for reflex and cognitive processes. Animal spirits arriving at the brain in sensory nerves were either reflected back down to the motor nerves of muscles to account for reflex behavior, such as withdraw of the hand from a painful stimulus, or the animal spirits made their way through the winding furrows of the cerebral cortex, producing complex thoughts and behavioral responses such as anguish or pleasure. Animal spirits transported in the nerves to the muscles did not inflate the muscles, as proposed by Descartes, but rather triggered a chemical reaction, "a type of explosion" that caused the muscle to contract [8]. Willis was an alchemist in addition to being a physician. In the book *Cerebri Anatome* (The

Anatomy of the Brain) published in 1664, Willis introduced the term "neurologie" to describe his "doctrine of the nerves."

In his book, Willis noted that the study of the nervous system "revealed the true and genuine reasons for very many of the actions and passions that take place in our body, which otherwise seem most difficult to explain: and from this fountain, no less than the hidden cases of diseases and symptoms, which are commonly ascribed to the incantations of witches, may be discovered and satisfactorily explained" [9]. In other words, hysteria and analogous disorders were rooted in the brain. Willis felt that the wandering uterus theory of antiquity was anatomically impossible and that the competing theory that vapors released during menstruation gravitated upward in the body were inconsistent with his observation that identical hysterical symptoms occurred in premenstrual and postmenopausal women. Furthermore, Willis observed that men often suffered from identical hysterical symptoms as women but the symptoms were given other names, such as hypochondriasis, and attributed to other causes such as obstruction of the spleen. Rather than the traditional treatments of body evacuations with bleeding, purging and vomiting, Willis recommended treating these patients with "flatteries" and "more gentle Physick" [10].

Hysteria, a Nervous Disorder

By the end of the seventeenth century, although traditional gynecological theories on hysteria remained engrained in the broad general practice of medicine, physicians in larger metropolitan areas and many of their affluent clientele accepted the "nervous" origin of the disorder. Terms such as hysteria and vapors in women and hypochondria and spleen in men were often used interchangeably to describe mild nervous disorders that needed to be distinguished from the more serious nervous disorders such as lunacy, insanity and severe melancholia. Sir Richard Blackmore, a prominent physician to royalty and affluent society in the early eighteenth century, wrote a book entitled *A Treatise of the Spleen and Vapours: Or Hypochondria and Hysterical Affection,s* in which he noted that "Vapours in women and Spleen in men is what neither sex are pleased to own" [11]. He emphasized that patients were reluctant to accept these diagnoses because many in the general public dismissed them as imaginary, but their pain and suffering were as real as that of any other patient. Blackmore recommended against aggressive treatments such as bleeding and purging for these nervous disorders but rather suggested calming medications like opium that would relax the patient and restore health. He further noted that many of these same patients suffered from anxiety and despondency, symptoms that were also helped by rest and sedating medications. No doubt, Blackmore's book was not only aimed at his fellow physicians but also at his highly educated affluent patients who were much more receptive to these mild treatments than the aggressive treatments provided by his competitors. Not unlike the current-day practice of medicine, physicians in the eighteenth century needed to be receptive to patients with psychogenic illness if they wanted to make a living.

Early Treatments of Hysteria

In the sixteenth century, the Swiss German philosopher, alchemist and physician Philippus von Hohenheim first introduced the European medical community to opium in the form of laudanum, a mixture of opium and wine for treating nervous disorders. Von Hohenheim, better known as Paracelsus, Latin for "equal to Celsus" (a well-known Roman physician), lectured in German rather than Latin so that common people could understand his ideas. In England, Thomas Sydenham used a laudanum preparation to treat hysteria and a wide range of nervous disorders. He noted that hysteria could mimic any organic disorder, including apoplexy, headaches with vomiting (migraine) and palpitations of the heart. Sydenham's laudanum consisted of opium dissolved in sherry wine with added saffron, cinnamon and clove. As the popularity of laudanum for treating nervous disorders rapidly spread addiction to laudanum became a major health issue in English society. Two of the many famous laudanum addicts were the fictional detective Sherlock Holmes and the Victorian author Thomas De Quincey, whose book *Confessions of an English Opium-Eater* is still considered one of the best books ever written on drug addiction.

Throughout the 18th and 19th centuries, patients with psychogenic disorders such as hysteria were the staple of medical practices throughout Europe, particularly in the larger cities such as London, Paris and Vienna, where the best physicians tended to gravitate. By attributing their patients' symptoms to nervous irritability and placing them in a somatic framework, physicians could justify regular visits and a range of treatments, particularly for affluent clientele. The stated goal of their treatments was to calm the nervous irritation. They used a range of drugs including bromides, opium, quinine, strychnine, arsenic and mercury. In America, Benjamin Rush, considered the father of American psychiatry and one of the original signers of the Declaration of Independence, believed that mental illness could cause somatic symptoms by altering brain circulation. In 1812, he published the first American textbook on mental diseases, *Medical Inquiries and Observations Upon the Diseases of the Mind,* in which he attempted to bridge the gap between psychiatry and general medicine [12]. In practice, Rush, who was Professor of Medicine at Philadelphia College, used a variety of treatments that would now be considered archaic and even cruel. For example, he championed the use of mercury in the form of calomel, noting that it removed the morbid excitement from the brain. Unfortunately, mercury is a toxin that can kill nerve cells, so the calming effect came at the price of losing nerve cells. Rush was the great bleeder. He bled everyone frequently and profusely, in some cases bleeding more than half of a patient's total blood volume. Rush's approach of purging and bloodletting epitomized the practice of medicine in America in the early nineteenth century.

Often medical treatments were augmented by recommendations for a visit to the sea or the mountains where the fresh sea and mountain air helped relieve the nervous irritability. In England, a trip to Bath for bathing in and drinking the sulfurous waters was popular. German spas, where physicians prescribed hot or cold baths and showers to calm the nervous irritation, were very popular for treating nervous disorders. Many still recommended flowing warm water and massages of the pelvis to stimulate the female genitals. So-called hydrotherapy did have its detractor, and many prominent European physicians considered it a form of quackery. Electrotherapy was another treatment for hysteria beginning in the mid-eighteenth century, but its heyday for treating psychogenic disorders didn't come until the late 19th and early 20th centuries. In the latter half of the eighteenth century, there were several reports of the use of a Leyden Jar, a portable device for storing and discharging sparks, to cure weakness and fatigue associated with hysteria. In America, the electricity enthusiast, Benjamin Franklin, claimed to cure a young woman with hysterical fits using a Leyden Jar. The first insight into how nerves really work came at the end of the eighteenth century when an Italian biologist, Luigi Galvani, serendipitously observed that he could make a frog's leg twitch by stimulating it with a pulse of electricity. He suggested that nerves generated electrical currents and that the muscle twitches he observed were caused by electricity, not "animal spirits." This was a revolutionary idea because, at the time, people believed that living organisms were governed by fundamentally different principles than inanimate objects. If electricity could activate nerves, then it might be useful for treating nervous disorders. By the late nineteenth century, large hospitals around the world had electricity departments with Leyden Jars and newly developed batteries that were used to apply electrical currents to different parts of the body, including the head.

Despite these different treatments, patients with hysteria rarely seemed to get better, often consulting many physicians if they could afford it. Not surprisingly, some developed animosity toward the medical profession. But physicians complained about having to deal with such chronic complaining patients who seemed determined to remain invalids. Many physicians believed that symptoms resulted either from a pathological process or fakery. There was no intermediate. As such they recommended a range of sadistic treatments for hysteria. W. Tyler Smith, a prominent English physician at the time, prescribed ice water into the rectum, ice in the vagina and leeches on the labia and cervix to treat the "nervous" menopausal women that filled his waiting room [13]. Other physicians recommended burning of the female genitals with caustic agents. Although these extreme treatments may have had some basis in early theories on the cause of hysteria, they also reflected the anger that many physicians felt towards women with this disorder. In 1853, another English physician, Robert Brudenell Carter, published a book entitled *On the Pathology and Treatments of Hysteria,* in which he speculated that although the initial hysterical fit might have been due to some pathological process, over time the process evolved into secondary and tertiary symptoms that were deliberately instituted by the patient [14]. In other words, Carter felt that hysterical patients were simulating illness. He felt that their symptoms were related to a prior illness, suggested by their physician or related to an illness witnessed in another person, but they were not real and deserved scorn. Unlike Smith, Carter felt that inflicting physical pain on these patients was useless, since they already were inflicting more pain on themselves than any physician could possibly prescribe. Carter suggested that physicians must overcome "the moral endurance of the patients" [15]. He should remain aloof and not show sympathy or alarm no matter how bad the symptoms. Carter recommended that the physician should employ "mental warfare" using humiliation, shame and threats of exposure to achieve a cure. "In all cases it will be necessary to use plain words, and to convey the idea of selfishness, and falsehood by their simplest names, and not under the disguise of any polite and elegant periphrasis" [16]. Carter also blamed the families of the hysterical patient, suggesting that they were often complacent in supporting the patient's convictions and interfered in his efforts to treat the patient. They couldn't believe that their lovely daughter was malingering. Carter's hard-line management of patients with hysteria is still engrained in sectors of the medical community, particularly in England. I have a strange sense of unease when I recall my time as an exchange medical student at St. Mary's Hospital in London in the mid-1960s. The senior neurological registrar, a professor Dr. Edwards, would see patients in his examining suite and we students would sit in and observe. If the patient's symptoms were at all suggestive of hysteria, we could tell because Dr. Edwards' neck veins would start to swell and his face turn red. As the examination proceeded, if Edwards became convinced of hysteria, he would become belligerent and berate the patient. On a few frightening occasions (for us students and the patient), he literally chased the patient out of the room, screaming "How dare you waste my valuable time?" As with other cures of the time, Carter and his followers claimed a high success rate for confrontational therapy, but there are no data to support the claim, and one might reasonably wonder whether by success he was referring to the fact that the patients rarely returned for a follow-up visit.

Spinal Irritation and the Spinal Reflex Theory

In the early nineteenth century, a senior physician at the Royal Infirmary in Glasgow, Thomas Brown, introduced the term "spinal irritation" to explain hysteria [17]. Excessive sensory stimulation caused spinal irritation and a range of sensory and motor symptoms, including dizziness, headaches, tics, paralysis and even fits. Brown searched for sensitive areas on the skin that might be the source of the spinal irritation and attacked them with blistering, leeches and cupping. In women, he felt that the uterine system provided a continuous source of spinal irritation that explained their "constitutional irritability." A natural offshoot of the spinal irritation theory was the spinal reflex theory of hysteria. The role of the spinal cord as a reflex center for the control of muscles and body organs was just beginning to be appreciated. Sensory signals originating from the skin and other body organs triggered reflex motor responses in the spinal cord. Since the spine was thought to be the main reflex center of the nervous system, nerves in the spine controlled all body organs and could produce symptoms at a subconscious level. The reflex theory also explained how diseases in one part of the body could affect other parts of the body. Because women's reproductive organs were thought to be most susceptible to irritation, they were the organs that triggered the most reflex responses causing symptoms throughout the body. Most physicians still felt that the uterus was the center of reflex pathology, not the wandering uterus of ancient times but rather a diseased or irritated uterus. Through spinal reflexes, it could influence all body organs, the heart, stomach, skin and eyes and ears. Ophthalmologists made the diagnosis of *kopiopia hysterica,* eyestrain of uterine origin. Indigestion and chest pain were blamed on uterine irritation. Reflexes could also spread to the brain and overcome reasoning causing a wide range of nervous symptoms. Andrew Scull facetiously summarized the androcentric nature of the spinal reflex theory in his book *Hysteria*: "Women, who possessed a large and complicated reproductive apparatus and only small brains, were thus far more susceptible than the male of the species to the predominance of reflex action over rational thought" [18].

Based on the spinal reflex theory, it was common to divide hysteria into two types, motor and sensory. Motor hysteria was characterized by a variety of motor symptoms, including paralysis, tics, muscle contractions and fits while sensory hysteria was manifested by sensory symptoms including pain, numbness and paresthesia, headache, dizziness and fatigue. Most patients exhibited both motor and sensory symptoms, but some would have just motor or sensory symptoms. As we will see, over time the symptom complex evolved from predominantly motor symptoms to predominantly sensory symptoms.

Two distinguished neurologists in the mid-nineteenth century, Moritz Romberg in Berlin and Charles Edouard Brown-Séquard in Paris, embraced the spinal reflex theory of hysteria to explain a range of symptoms seen in their patients [19]. Romberg is best known for the neurological test named after him in which a patient stands with feet together first with eyes open and then closed. Loss of balance with eye closure suggests loss of peripheral sensation such as occurs with peripheral neuropathy. In Romberg's time, the test was most useful for identifying tabes dorsalis, a variant of neurosyphylis that selectively involved the sensory tracts at the back of the spinal cord (the dorsal columns). Like many others, Romberg thought that both men and women were susceptible to hysteria but it was more common in women because their reproductive organs were in a constant state of irritation, whereas men's reproductive organs were more stable. In women, menses and pregnancy increased irritability and could trigger an attack. Romberg used local treatments on the uterine system to reduce excitability and recommended rest and baths to decrease reflex nervous excitability. He also counseled women to resist their bodily impulses, i.e., masturbation. He felt that masturbation bombarded the spinal cord with nerve impulses triggering reflex sensory and motor activity. He set the stage for later more aggressive treatments aimed at preventing masturbation.

Brown-Séquard was born in Paris in 1818, the son of an American father and French mother. After his medical training in Paris he taught at Harvard Medical School and practiced neurology in New York and London before returning to Paris to succeed Claude Bernard as Professor of Experimental Medicine at the College of France. Early in his career, he focused on the sensory and motor pathways in the spinal cord first in guinea pigs and then in patients. Cutting the right half of the spinal cord in guinea pigs caused a loss of muscle function in the right leg and loss of pain and temperature sensation in the left leg. He concluded that the pain and temperature signals crossed after entering the spinal cord and ran on the opposite side. Later he described detailed studies on patients with spinal cord damage where he precisely mapped the loss of sensation to pain, warmth, cold and touch and argued that each sensation ascended in different tracts in the spinal cord. The neurological sign of weakness in one leg and loss of pain and temperature sensation in the opposite leg (the Brown-Séquard sign) is still a reliable indicator of damage to half of the spinal cord (on the side of the weakness). Based on the spinal reflex theory, Brown-Séquard performed detailed examinations of the skin in his patients with hysteria looking for trigger points for their symptoms. Once the trigger points were identified, he would burn the skin over these areas with a cotton cone soaked in a combustible substance, called moxa. Often the pain was so intense with this treatment that the patient would scream in agony, and many suffered severe burns that took months to heal.

Brown-Séquard added a new twist to the reflex theory of hysteria when in a series of articles in the English journal *Lancet* he argued that irritated and diseased nerves produced secretions that entered the blood stream and affected distant organs including the brain [20]. He felt that nerves from the genito-urinary organs were particularly susceptible to producing secretions that traveled throughout the body, causing symptoms from pain to indigestion. If the secretions traveled to the brain, they could cause a range of nervous disorders from hysteria to insanity. All of these terrible nervous disorders might result from just a slight irritation of a pelvic nerve. Brown-Séquard made quite a stir at age 72 when he claimed to have discovered the fountain of youth by injecting himself with fluid derived from the testicles of freshly killed guinea pigs and dogs. He survived the injections but died of natural causes a few years later.

The Attack on the Female Genitalia

Although neurologists and their theories on hysteria in the mid-nineteenth century did pose a threat to the female genito-urinary system, their treatments were relatively mild compared with other subspecialists. Psychiatrists (called alienists or asylum superintendents at the time) saw female masturbation as having a pivotal role in hysteria and insanity. This theory led to a range of treatments from burning with a hot iron to the application of a variety of caustic agents on the female genitals in an effort to discourage the "filthy habit." Even these sadistic treatments paled in comparison to the attack on the female genitals made by the newly developing subspecialty of gynecology. The great majority of these men believed that the pelvic organs of their patients were causing havoc with their emotional health. Furthermore, they convinced their patients that their pelvic organs were toxic and needed to be removed.

A leading gynecologist in England, Isaac Baker Brown, dismissed other efforts to discourage masturbation as halfway measures and recommended going right to the seat of the problem and remove the woman's clitoris. Baker Brown, who was known for his surgical skills, was the first to use chloroform in childbirth and for gynecological operations. With the publication of *Surgical Diseases of Women* in 1854, he established himself as a preeminent gynecologist and was later elected President of the Medical Society of London. In a later book, Baker Brown assured his readers that masturbation initiated spinal irritation, causing hysteria, fits, idiocy, mania and eventually death [21]. He justified his extreme treatment as the only way to prevent the nervous exhaustion caused by masturbation. To remove the clitoris, Baker Brown seized it with a set of curved forceps and moved the edge of a red-hot iron around the base. He bragged that he had never had a case that he couldn't cure with this procedure [22]. Baker Brown not only publicized his operation to his fellow physicians but to the lay public as well. An article in the *Church Times* endorsed his operation and urged clergymen to recommend the procedure to their parishioners [23]. This procedure was largely abandoned in the latter part of the nineteenth century in Europe, but it remained popular in America well into the twentieth century.

Moritz Romberg not only set the stage for the gynecological attack on the clitoris but he was also instrumental in focusing attention on the ovaries. He claimed that he could trigger a hysterical fit by pressing on the ovaries simply by placing his hand over the lower abdomen and pushing downward [24]. Subsequently, physicians in Europe and America claimed to start or stop hysterical attacks with pressure on the ovaries and, as we will see, even the great French neurologist, Charcot, regularly applied pressure to the ovaries in his female patients as part of his examination. Because hysterical symptoms were thought to be more common around the time of menses, the notion of reflex ovarian hysteria made sense. Ovarian ablations were first routinely performed for a variety of diseases in the mid-nineteenth century but the first ovarian ablation for treating hysteria was performed in 1872 by an American gynecologist Robert Battey in Rome, Georgia [25]. His patient, a young single woman suffering from a range of hysterical symptoms from headaches to fits, developed sepsis after the surgery but eventually recovered, and Battey claimed that all of her nervous symptoms disappeared. A colleague of Battey suggested that the operation be called Battey's operation, and his fellow gynecologists frequently used the phrase "to Batteyise a woman," which meant to take out normal ovaries to treat a nervous disorder. The operation rapidly spread to Europe, particularly England and Germany, but it made little inroads in France because of Charcot's opposition. In America, more ovarian ablations were performed for nervous disorders than for treating diseases of the ovaries by the end of the nineteenth century. The operation was still being performed well into the mid-twentieth century.

One might reasonably ask why would women allow their physicians to perform such brutal procedures on their reproductive organs? The answer is more complicated than simply misogyny, which no doubt did play a role. The physicians truly believed in the reflex theory of hysteria and so did the lay public, particularly members of the affluent class who could afford to pay for these expensive procedures. In many instances, women would demand that their physicians perform a surgical procedure for their intolerable symptoms. These women knew that their symptoms were "not just in their head," as they were often told. Having a diagnosis and undergoing a surgical procedure confirmed to their friends and families that their symptoms were "real." Even more remarkable, although female physicians were rare at the time, a few prominent female physicians in America endorsed the use of ovarian ablation for treating nervous disorders in women. Most physicians were beginning to accept the fact that hysterical symptoms could also occur in men, but castration in men was rarely performed to treat the symptoms. Were the predominantly male physicians uneasy about mutilating the genitals in patients of their own gender? It seems likely. At the turn of the twentieth century, Archibald Church, a prominent neurologist at Northwestern University in Illinois, noted "Men do not accept mutilating operations upon the genital tract with the equanimity which is presented by the gentler sex, who peaceably accept unsexing operations without much question as to their effect, provided they can be relieved of some trivial or temporary ailment" [26].

In the latter part of the nineteenth century, proponents of the spinal reflex theory, particularly in the newly developed subspecialty of rhinology, suggested that the nasal mucosa was reflexively connected to other body organs so that diseases of different organs could be treated nasally. The basic thinking was that the trigeminal nerve, the main sensory nerve of the nose and face, was interconnected with nerves to other organs through its brainstem nucleus. In 1884, John Mackenzie, a surgeon at the Baltimore Ear, Nose and Throat Hospital, proposed that the genitals and nose had a particularly strong influence on each other [27]. To support his contention, he noted that the nasal mucosa can swell during menstruation and that nosebleeds might replace menstruation. He quoted earlier reports that in men the size of the nose and the penis corresponded, and there was histological similarity between the erectile tissue of the nose and penis. Mackenzie warned that irritation of the nose causes irritation of the genitals and that frequent masturbation could cause nasal problems. Nasal cautery and nasal douches soon became popular treatments for a wide range of nervous disorders in both women and men. In Berlin, a prominent general practitioner and friend of Sigmund Freud, Wilhelm Fliess, claimed to have identified a genital site on the nasal mucosa and proceeded to treat female symptoms by dabbing cocaine on the site [28]. Sigmund Freud later had his nasal mucosa cauterized for a variety of psychosomatic symptoms.

Hysteria and Fasting Girls

There is a long and fascinating history of fasting young women who refuse to eat food [29]. As with other early manifestations of hysteria, such fasting was initially thought to result from possession by supernatural spirits and treated accordingly, but later fasting became recognized as a common symptom in hysteria. A nun in thirteenth century Leicester, England was said to have fasted for 7 years with her only nourishment being the Holy Eucharist, which she received every Sunday. Hugh, Bishop of Lincoln, declared the young woman authentic after he sent 15 clerks to monitor her every activity for 15 days, never letting her out of their sight. They confirmed that she ingested no food yet maintained good strength and health. Numerous saints, including Saint Catharine of Sienna, Saint Rose of Lima and Saint Collete of Alcantara were said to live only on sacramental bread. Saint Prosper of Aquitaine described a young girl possessed by the devil who hadn't eaten for 70 days yet maintained her health and vigor. He claimed that every night at midnight the devil sent a bird to provide her with nourishment. Many of the fasting young women thought to be possessed by the devil also complained of gastrointestinal symptoms such as abdominal pain and rigidity and a "lump in the throat" suggestive of classical globus hystericus. In 1595, the famous Italian anatomist and surgeon Fabricius examined a 13-year-old girl whose parents claimed she had lived for 3 years without any food or drink; their claims were backed by testimony from a variety of public officials. He noted a melancholy countenance but overall normal appearance except for her abdomen, which was compressed and appeared to cleave to her back-bone. Her liver and bowels were hardened to the touch, and she did not produce any excrement or urine. She abhorred any kind of food and if someone tried to place food in her mouth she swooned away. Despite the lack of nourishment, Fabricius marveled at her ability to dance and play with other children. Around the same time, a young Dutch woman from Meurs was said to have fasted for 14 years, 1597 to 1611, from age 21 to age 36, confirmed by testimony from magistrates of Meurs and a minister who had her stay at his house for 13 days where she was carefully watched but took no food. Her story was immortalized in a Latin verse:

> Meursæ hæc quam cernis decies ter, sexque peregit,
> Annos, bis septem prorsus non viscitur annis.
> Nec potat, sic sola sedet, sic pallida vitam.
> Ducit, et exigui se oblectat floribus horti [30].
> [This maid of Meurs thirty and six years spent,
> Fourteen of which she took no nourishment;
> Thus pale and wan she sits sad and alone,
> A garden's all she loves to look upon.]

In the nineteenth century with the emphasis on scientific medicine, people became more skeptical of reports of prolonged fasting. Ann Moore, a young woman from Staffordshire, England, claimed she had not eaten food for 6 years since she had washed the linen of a woman with ulcers over her body [31]. Ann became nauseated with the mere sight of food, and she was obviously emaciated. To confirm her claim, she agreed to be watched by a group of volunteers for 3 weeks, and they provided testimony that she took no nourishment during that time. As Ann's fame spread, people came from all over England, leaving donations of several hundred pounds. But skeptics remained, and she agreed to a second observation, this time including a prominent local physician and his son. Ann was weighed daily, showing that she was gradually losing weight; by the ninth day she was emaciated, and the doctor told her she would die if she continued the experiment. She finally admitted that she had been eating secretively over the past 6 years and that during the initial observation she had contrived with her daughter to bring her towels soaked with milk and gravy and to convey food from mouth to mouth when kissing her daughter. Dr. John Ogle at St. George's Hospital in London described a 20-year-old woman who had been hospitalized for months with hysteria who refused to eat any kind of food and if made to eat would immediately vomit. By chance an employee found a note addressed to a fellow patient: "Dear Mrs. Evens,—I was very sorry you should take the trouble of cutting me such a nice piece of bread and butter, yesterday. I would of taken it but all of them saw you send it, and then they would have made enough to have talked about. But I should be very glad if you would cut me a nice piece of crust and put it in a piece of paper and send it, or else bring it, so that they do not see it, for they all watch me very much, and I should like to be your friend and you to be mine. Mrs. Winslow, (the nurse) is going to chapel. I will make it up with you when I can go as far. Do not send it if you cannot spare it. Goodbye, and God bless you" [32]. Although she initially denied writing the note, she eventually confessed and left the hospital.

The best documented and the most talked about case of prolonged fasting in the nineteenth century was that of Sarah Jacob, the "Welsh Fasting Girl." Dr. Robert Fowler, an Edinburgh physician, became interested in the case and wrote a small book documenting the facts in 1871 [33]. Sarah, said to be a very pretty child given to religious reading, was the intelligent daughter of simple Welsh farmers. At age 10, she began complaining of belly pain and soon after had her first hysterical fit. During the fit she developed the classical reverse C position of the body so that only the head and heels touched the bed. Once the muscle spasm stopped, she would fall full length onto the bed. For the next month she had repeated fits and took little food. She then had periods of unresponsiveness followed by sudden awakenings and the parents reported that the small amount of food she was given was regurgitated. Bowel movements were rare, and she spent all of her time in bed. By the tenth of October 1867 it was declared that she stopped taking any food and only occasional small amounts of water. The parents vehemently held to their claim that she took no food and that even the mention of food made her excited and could trigger a fit. A local vicar and several nurses provided testimonials that she took no food. But others were skeptical and warned the parents that it was physically impossible to survive without nourishment and that other similar cases were eventually proven fraudulent. But the parents were convinced it was a miracle. Their child was cared for by the "Big Doctor," the "God Almighty." As with other similar cases, the child became well known and people came from near and far, leaving money and gifts, particularly fine clothes. The "wonderful girl living without food" was elaborately dressed for the visiting pilgrims and her health improved despite the lack of nourishment. Other than a few skeptics, the lay community was convinced of the child's veracity as documented by a letter to a local newspaper in February 1869:

> To the Editor of the Welshman.
> "Sir: Allow me to invite the attention of your readers to a most extraordinary case. Sarah Jacob, a little girl twelve years of age, and daughter of Mr. Evan Jacob, Lletherneuadd, in this parish, has not partaken of a single grain of any kind of food whatever, during the last sixteen months. She did occasionally swallow a few drops of water during the first few months of this period; but now she does not even do that. She still looks pretty well in the face and continues in the possession of all her mental faculties. She is in this and several other respects, a wonderful little girl. Medical men persist in saying that the thing is quite impossible, but all the nearest neighbors, who are thoroughly acquainted with the circumstances of the case, entertain no doubt whatever of the subject, and I am myself of the same opinion. Would it not be worth their while for medical men to make an investigation into the

nature of this strange case? Mr. Evan Jacob would readily admit into his house any respectable person who might be anxious to watch it and to see for himself. I may add, that Lletherneuadd is a farm-house about a mile from New Inn, in this parish.

Yours faithfully,

THE VICAR OF LLANFIHANGEL-AR-ARTH" [34].

Based on this letter from the vicar, the community organized a public meeting and decided to organize a committee of volunteer watchers to monitor the young girl for 2 weeks to prove that she was not eating. The watchers were neighborhood gentlemen who took alternating 12-hour shifts watching Sarah to be sure she was not ingesting food. All seven watchers, including three prior skeptics, provided statements that Sarah did not eat anything during their watch but when later questioned it was obvious that the watch was imperfect, since some left before their observation period ended and several were drinking alcohol and one was actually drunk during the watch. Regardless, after the watch report, Sarah's reputation grew and larger crowds came to visit.

It was in this circus-like atmosphere that Dr. Fowler first visited Sarah on August 30, 1869. As he exited the train, he saw young boys carrying signs saying "Fasting Girl" and "This is the shortest way to Llethernoryadd-ucha" [35]. As he entered the child's room he noted: "The child was lying on a bed decorated as a bride, having around her head a wreath of flowers, from which was suspended a smart ribbon, the ends of which were joined by a small bunch of flowers, after the present fashion of ladies' bonnet strings…Her face was plump, and her cheeks and lips of a beautiful rosy color. Her eyes were bright and sparkling, the pupils were very dilated, in a measure explicable by the fact of the child's head and face being shaded from the windowlight by the projecting side of the cupboard bedstead. There was that restless movement and frequent looking out at the corners of the eyes so characteristic of simulative disease. Considering the lengthened inactivity of the girl, her muscular development was very good, and the amount of fat layer not inconsiderable" [36]. When Fowler examined the child, she complained of pain when touched and she had a brief period of hysterical crying and sobbing that her mother called a fit. Fowler found her examination to be rather unremarkable with normal bowel sounds despite the fact that the parents stated that she had not had any food for the past 23 months. In a letter to the *London Times* Fowler concluded: "The whole case is in fact one of simulative hysteria, in a young girl having the propensity to deceive very strongly developed. Therewith may be probably associated the power or habit of prolonged fasting. Both patient and mother admitted the occasional occurrence of the choking sensation called globus hystericus" [37].

Not surprisingly, this letter to the *Times* reinvigorated public interest in the case, and after a second public meeting it was decided to bring in a group of trained nurses from Guy's Hospital in London to conduct a second watching but this time with a carefully thought out plan to prevent any possible trickery. The experienced nurses were told to allow her to have food if she asked for it but to be sure she did not get any food without their knowledge. The watch began on December 9, 1869 and the child began to gradually deteriorate and by December 16th, the nurses became extremely concerned and told the parents that the child was dying and the watch must be stopped. The parents refused, saying she had been like this before and it wasn't due to her not eating. Sarah died the next day. There was immediate public outcry and a coroner's inquest concluded that the child died of starvation and that the father was to blame and guilty of manslaughter. In a subsequent trial, both the father and mother were found guilty of manslaughter, with the father getting 12 months of prison at hard labor and the wife 6 months. It was determined that no case could be made against the physicians who advised the nurses but did not take part in the watch.

In America, a well-known case of a fasting young woman in Brooklyn, New York became famous worldwide when an article was published in the New York Herald in October 1878, "Life without Food. An Invalid Lady who for fourteen years has lived without nourishment" [38]. The unique features of this case were that the young woman, Miss Mollie Fancher, had been involved in an accident that apparently damaged her spinal cord, since she was paralyzed in the legs, but she had typical symptoms of hysteria and also claimed to be a clairvoyant and spiritualist. Unlike other cases, Mollie's parents were reclusive and did not seek attention, and several local doctors, including the woman's family doctor, a Dr. Speir, supported her claim that she did not eat any food for years. The case developed notoriety when Dr. William Hammond, one of the founding fathers of American Neurology and the Surgeon General during the civil war, wrote a letter to the Herald challenging the possibility that a person could survive without food and offering a thousand dollars to the young woman or the charity of her choice if she and her family would permit a group of neurologists to watch her for a few weeks to confirm that she was not consuming any food [39]. Having been well aware of the case of Sarah Jacob, Dr. Hammond stipulated that they would work with the family doctor and if the doctor saw signs of deteriorating health, they would force her to eat to save her life. Dr. Hammond, who had written extensively on starving young girls, was also very interested in clairvoyance and spiritualism and noted in his letter that her claims of mind reading were "humbug." The young girl and her family did not respond to Dr. Hammond's challenge.

One of the key questions regarding these fasting young women is whether they were intentionally trying to deceive their physicians and the lay public. Several of them were eventually shown to be secretly ingesting food, and it is physically impossible to survive without nourishment for more than a few weeks. Dr. Hammond noted that hysterical patients did have a remarkable ability to go without food for long periods of time and that he had seen patients fast from 1 to 11 days but beyond that time symptoms became unbearable and the patients invariably broke their fast. With regard to whether Mollie Fancher was intentionally trying to deceive, Hammond argued: "Hysteria is a disease as much beyond the control of the patient as inflammation of the brain or any other disease. A proclivity to simulation and deception is just as much a symptom of hysteria as pain is of pleurisy. To say, therefore, that she simulated abstinence and deceived us to the quantity of food she took, is no imputation on her honesty, or questioning her possession of as high a degree of honor and trust, as can be claimed by any one. Other women naturally as moral as she, have under the influence of hysteria perpetrated the grossest deceptions, and they are not unfrequently manifested in the very same way that hers apparently are. Her case is by no means an isolated one; it is not such as has never been seen before; it does not 'knock the bottom out of all existing medical theories, and is in a word miraculous,' as one of the physicians is reported to have said" [40]. Are these fasting young women with hysteria the same as modern young women with anorexia nervosum? There are similarities in the single-minded determination to avoid food and nausea and regurgitation if forced to eat, but the motivation for fasting with anorexia nervosum is typically a distorted body image with concerns about being overweight, whereas with hysteria it is gastrointestinal symptoms such as abdominal pain and discomfort and a lump in the throat (globus hystericus).

In Brief

Early theories on the cause of hysteria evolved from ancient ideas of a wandering uterus and vapors to medieval beliefs in evil spirits and the supernatural to early nineteenth century ideas of spinal reflex irritation activated by excessive sensory signals originating from the female reproductive organs. Symptoms ranged from paralysis, bizarre behaviors and fits to fasting, abdominal pain and difficulty swallowing to generalized pain, fatigue and dizziness. Treatments focused on the female reproductive organs, ranging from advice to increase sexual activity and decrease masturbation to surgical ablation of the clitoris, uterus or ovaries. With the development of scientific medicine in the nineteenth century, these early theories were questioned and even ridiculed. Regardless, many of these ancient misogynistic concepts still pervade the public perception of hysteria.

References

1. Scull A. Hysteria: the disturbing history. New York: Oxford University Press; 2009. p. 11.
2. Rousseau G. A strange pathology: hysteria in the early modern world. In: Gilman SL, King H, Porter R, et al. Hysteria beyond Freud. Berkeley: University of California Press; 1993.
3. Scull A. Hysteria: the disturbing history. New York: Oxford University Press; 2009. p. 12–25.
4. Maines R. The technology of orgasm: "hysteria," the vibrator and Women's sexual satisfaction. Baltimore: Johns Hopkins University Press; 1999.
5. Waller J. A forgotten plague: making sense of dance mania. Lancet. 2009;373:624–5.
6. MacDonald M (ed. and intro.). Witchcraft and hysteria in Elizabethan London, Edward Jorden and the Mary Glover case. London: Routledge/Tavistock; 1991.
7. Schiff S. The Witches of Salem. The New Yorker 2015 September 7.
8. Zimmer C. Soul made flesh: the discovery of the brain – and how it changed the world. New York: Free Press; 2004.
9. Willis T. Cerebri anatome. London: Royal College of Surgeons of England; 1664. p. 124.
10. Willis T. An essay on the pathology of the brain and nervous stock. London: Dring, Harper and Leigh; 1681.
11. Blackmore R. A treatise of the spleen and Vapours: or, Hypochondriacal and hysterical affections, vol. 1726. London: Pemberton. p. 97.
12. Rush B. Medical inquiries and observations upon the diseases of the mind. 5th ed. Philadelphia: Gregg and Eliot; 1835.

13. Smith WT. The climacteric disease of women. Lond J Med. 1848;1:607.
14. Brudenell Carter R. On the pathology and treatment of hysteria. London: Churchill; 1853.
15. Brudenell Carter R. On the pathology and treatment of hysteria. London: Churchill; 1853. p. 108.
16. Brudenell Carter R. On the pathology and treatment of hysteria. London: Churchill; 1853. p. 114.
17. Brown T. On irritation of the spinal nerves. Glasgow Med J. 1828;1:131–60.
18. Scull A. Hysteria: the disturbing history. New York: Oxford University Press; 2009. p. 73.
19. Shorter E. From paralysis to fatigue: a history of psychosomatic illness in the modern era. New York: Free Press; 1992. p. 42–6.
20. Brown-Séquard E. Course of lectures on the physiology and pathology of the central nervous system. Lancet. 1858;ii:519–20.
21. Baker Brown I. On the curability of certain forms of insanity, epilepsy, catalepsy, and hysteria in females. London: Hardwicke; 1866.
22. Scull A. Hysteria: the disturbing history. New York: Oxford University Press; 2009. p. 79.
23. Scull A. Hysteria: the disturbing history. New York: Oxford University Press; 2009. p. 7981.
24. Shorter E. From paralysis to fatigue: a history of psychosomatic illness in the modern era. New York: Free Press; 1992. p. 43.
25. Shorter E. From paralysis to fatigue: a history of psychosomatic illness in the modern era. New York: Free Press; 1992. p. 75.
26. Shorter E. From paralysis to fatigue: a history of psychosomatic illness in the modern era. New York: Free Press; 1992. p. 93.
27. MacKenzie JN. Irritation of the sexual apparatus as an etiological factor in the production of nasal disease. Am J Med Sci. 1884;87:360–5.
28. Sulloway FJ. Freud: biologist of the mind. New York: Basic Books; 1979.
29. Hammond WA. Fasting girls: their physiology and pathology. New York: GP Putman's Sons; 1879.
30. Hammond WA. Fasting girls: their physiology and pathology, vol. 1879. New York: GP Putman's Sons. p. 9.
31. Hammond WA. Fasting girls: their physiology and pathology, vol. 11. New York: GP Putman's Sons; 1879. p. 12.
32. Hammond WA. Fasting girls: their physiology and pathology, vol. 1879. New York: GP Putman's Sons. p. 13.
33. Fowler R. Complete history of the case of the welsh fasting girl. London: Henry Renshaw; 1871.
34. Fowler R. Complete history of the case of the welsh fasting girl. London: Henry Renshaw; 1871. p. 15,16.
35. Fowler R. Complete history of the case of the welsh fasting girl, vol. 1871. London: Henry Renshaw. p. 29.
36. Fowler R. Complete history of the case of the welsh fasting girl. London: Henry Renshaw; 1871. p. 30.
37. Fowler R. Complete history of the case of the welsh fasting girl. London: Henry Renshaw; 1871. p. 31,32.
38. Hammond WA. Fasting girls: their physiology and pathology, vol. 1879. New York: GP Putman's Sons. p. 49.
39. Hammond WA. Fasting girls: their physiology and pathology, vol. 1879. New York: GP Putman's Sons. p. 75.
40. Hammond WA. Fasting girls: their physiology and pathology, vol. 1879. New York: GP Putman's Sons. p. 57.

The Golden Age of Hysteria

3

> The nineteenth century was hysteria's golden age because it was then that the moral presence of the doctor became normative as never before in regulating intimate lives.
>
> Roy Porter [1].

The nineteenth century marked a gradual evolution from traditional to scientific medicine. Ancient concepts such a "humors" and "vital forces" were replaced with new concepts based on empirical measurements. Many of the active ingredients in herbal medications were isolated and entirely new drugs were synthesized. Vague medical diagnoses, such as "dropsy" and "fever," were replaced by more specific diagnoses with detailed clinical profiles and postmortem examinations. As the importance of the brain in overall health and disease became apparent, a new sub-specialty, neurology, developed. For the first time, the clinical features of neurological diseases such as stroke, multiple sclerosis and epilepsy were described in large series of patients. Nineteenth-century neurologists played a key role in redefining hysteria.

Briquet's Syndrome

The English physicians Thomas Willis and Thomas Sydenham had previously suggested that hysteria was a brain disorder that could affect both men and women, but this notion did not gain wider acceptance until the publication of *Treatise on Hysteria* by the French physician Paul Briquet in 1859 [2]. In his book, Briquet described the clinical and epidemiological features of patients with hysteria seen at the La Charité hospital in Paris over a 10-year period. Briquet defined hysteria as a "neurosis of the brain" that could affect children and men as well as women [3]. He was bothered by the misogynistic connotations of the word but he argued that hysteria had been generally accepted since the time of Hippocrates and that hopefully with time it would lose its pejorative implications. Ironically, more recently some

R. W. Baloh, *Medically Unexplained Symptoms*,
https://doi.org/10.1007/978-3-030-59181-6_3

have suggested replacing the term hysteria with "Briquet's syndrome" to avoid the negative connotations [4]. Despite providing several fully documented cases of hysteria in men, Briquet emphasized that the disorder was much more common in women. On reviewing the hospital records he found that 1000 women and only 50 men were diagnosed with hysteria; in his sample women were 20 times more likely to develop hysteria than men. When he surveyed the women patients in the hospital at any given time, he found that about 25% had a diagnosis of hysteria and another 25% were highly susceptible to developing hysteria meaning that they were emotionally labile. He explained this remarkably high percentage of female patients with or susceptible to hysteria based on the female temperament. "Amongst women there exists a more lively sensitiveness than amongst men. Feelings are more easily aroused, are experienced more intensely and have more repercussions in the whole economy than amongst men" [5]. Conflicting with the traditional view of hysteria as a disease of middle-aged women, Briquet found that 20% of patients with hysteria had onset before puberty and more than half had onset before the age of 20. This observation becomes even more important when one considers the overall poor prognosis in these patients; Briquet noted that "one quarter never recover or have the illness their entire life... Some young girls who became hysteric before the age of 12 or 13 years are condemned to a lifetime of suffering, malaise, and sometimes serious illnesses. They are always sick, abort easily, or if they go to term, give birth to more hysterics. Some remain ill until an advanced age, become cachectic, thin and irritable, and old before their time, leading but a wretched life for themselves and those around them" [6]. Briquet provided the first convincing evidence for a major inherited component to hysteria. He compared the incidence of hysteria in first degree relatives (parents, siblings and children) of patients in the hospital with hysteria and sick patients without hysteria and found that about 25% of relatives of patients with hysteria had hysteria, whereas only about 2% of relatives of patients without hysteria had hysteria. When just looking at the daughters of sick women, daughters of women with hysteria were 12 times more likely to have hysteria than daughters of sick women without hysteria.

Briquet identified what he considered a unique "moral disposition" of women who were at high risk of developing hysteria. As a child "they were extremely impressionable, very fearful, had a great fear of being scolded, and when they were choked, burst into tears, and ran away. When older, they experienced intense feelings for the slightest reason, cried when they heard a moving story, were extremely timid; they were afraid of everything" [7]. Men with these characteristics were also susceptible to developing hysteria. A life of maltreatment and suffering predisposed to developing hysteria. Contrary to prior reports, Briquet concluded that hysteria was more common in the lower classes than upper classes because the former had more difficult lives. "Joy, happiness and physical and morale pleasure never provoked hysteria, whereas grief, worry and sadness, jealousy, fear and apprehension most strongly predispose to hysteria" [8]. With regard to the role of sexual activity in predisposing to developing hysteria, he compared the incidence of hysteria in three groups – nuns, house servants and prostitutes – and found the highest incidence of hysteria in prostitutes, which he attributed to their difficult lives rather than to sexual overactivity. Contrary to the prevailing notion that young women with hysteria should marry, he provided several examples where women first developed hysteria after marriage and the symptoms stopped after death of their husband.

Briquet carefully documented the broad spectrum of symptoms associated with hysteria. He divided the symptoms into hyperaesthesias, anesthesias, perversions of sensation, spasms, seizures, paralysis, and abnormalities of muscle contraction, respiration and secretion. He emphasized "Pain in the muscles is so common that there is not a single woman with this neurosis who does not have some muscle pain during the course of the illness" [9]. He noted that areas of anesthesia (numbness) typically followed bizarre patterns and any of the primary sensations including vision, smell and touch could be distorted. He provided a detailed discussion of how to distinguish hysterical seizures from epileptic seizures and as Charcot would later emphasize, Briquet noted the role of imitation in producing seizures, "in my wards, the patient who has the strongest seizures gives the tone to the others" [10]. Overall, Briquet provided the most detailed clinical description of hysteria in the 19th century.

Charcot and His Hysterical Circus

Heavily influenced by Briquet's work on hysteria, Jean-Martin Charcot, the most famous neurologist of the latter half of the 19th century, also believed that hysteria was not a disease of the female reproductive organs but rather a brain disease that could affect men and women. To him the only difference between hysteria and other brain diseases was that the pathology of hysteria was yet to be found. Charcot was a thoughtful clinician and scientist whose name is attached to several neurological disorders yet as we will see in many ways his work on hysteria blemished an otherwise brilliant career.

The son of a wagon-maker, Charcot took advantage of Napoleon's merit-based education system to rapidly rise up through the medical hierarchy. After completing his medical training, he received an appointment at the Salpêtrière, a public hospital for destitute women on the outskirts of Paris. Patients at the Saltpêtrière represented a "museum" of neurological pathology. Some of them spent their life in the institute. Charcot applied the revolutionary new approach of clinical-pathological correlation to the study of neurological diseases. The patient's symptoms and signs observed prior to death were correlated with the findings at postmortem examination. Charcot and his students carefully documented symptoms and signs over decades and since most of his patients were poor and friendless, postmortem examinations were assured. A few of the many diseases that he personally described include: multiple sclerosis (which he called disseminated sclerosis), amyotrophic lateral sclerosis (often called Charcot's disease but in America called Lou Gehrig's disease after the New York Yankee baseball player who died of the disease) and the most common inherited neuropathy, now called Charcot-Marie-Toothe disease. Charcot became so prominent in neurological circles that no one questioned his diagnoses. If Charcot made a diagnosis the matter was settled. But his foray into the study of hysteria would change all that.

Like many of their British counterparts, some French physicians at the time believed that hysterical women were malingerers who deserved the disgust and condemnation of the medical profession. By contrast Charcot believed strongly that hysteria was an organic disease rooted in the brain. The fact that he was not able to identify a specific pathology with hysteria was not that surprising to him since at the time he could not find a specific pathology for other neurologic diseases such as epilepsy and chorea. Presumably there were diseases of the nervous system that left no material trace in the postmortem brain. Of course, his primitive microscopes limited his ability to identify such traces.

Charcot felt that the characteristic symptoms and signs of hysteria developed in someone with an underlying inherited susceptibility, "an inherent weakness" [11]. The idea of a familial disposition in patients with hysteria was not new but the suggestion of a genetic susceptibility was a new wrinkle. Charcot believed that the inherent weakness predisposed the patient to triggers such as physical or emotional trauma or even the presence of another person with hysteria. He had previously observed that when hysterical patients were housed on the same ward with epileptic patients the hysterical patients often developed epileptic-like fits. Thus, hysterical symptoms might travel from susceptible patient to susceptible patient causing an outbreak of hysteria (mass hysteria). Like all neurologists it was inevitable that Charcot would see many patients with hysteria in his general practice outside the hospital and he felt that he could make a diagnosis on the basis of characteristic symptoms and signs. Charcot primarily worked with women and felt that hysteria was more common in women but he did see men with identical symptoms. In women, he noted that ovarian tenderness was a common physical finding and applying pressure on the ovaries could trigger or modify their symptoms. In men, squeezing the testicles could have the same effect [12]. This observation seems a bit odd considering his premise that hysteria was a brain disease but he considered some type of interaction between the genitals and the brain, either neural or chemical that could trigger hysteria. The spinal reflex theory was still engrained in medical thinking.

Just as he had done with his other neurological disorders, Charcot along with his assistants described what they felt was a pathognomonic symptom pattern of a hysterical fit ("la grande hystérie") [13]. He identified four stages: (1) the epileptic phase manifested by jerking of the extremities, (2) the grand movement phase in which the patient developed bizarre contortions (such as the reverse C postures exhibited by Mary Glover) and vocal outbursts, (3) the passion phase in which the patient posed as if being in religious or erotic ecstasy, and (4) the delirium phase manifested by hallucinations and delusions. Although this presumed stereotypic pattern of symptoms and signs was used by Charcot to support his contention that hysteria was an organic disease of the brain, more likely the pattern resulted from overly zealous assistants and the eager to please patients. Whether Charcot himself was aware of these biases is unclear but he routinely demonstrated the different phases at his Tuesday rounds.

Charcot moved from the field of clinical science to the theatrical with his weekly hysteric "circus." Initially, these were simply medical rounds attended by fellow physicians and students but as Charcot's fame and fortune spiraled, his rounds became well known throughout affluent Parisian society. Writers, artists, academics, businessmen, and royalty alike attended the rounds during which Charcot displayed lightly clad young women with hysteria performing bizarre contortions and behaviors. With razor-sharp focus on his scientific mission, Charcot paraded these young women before the lay audience like animals in a circus tent, apparently oblivious to any pain and anguish they may have suffered. Many patients returned on a regular basis for Charcot's rounds; some became stars in Parisian society. Blanche Wittman, known as Charcot's pet hysteric and the queen of hysterics, was made famous in an 1887 painting by the French academic history painter, André Brouillet. In this painting, which captures Charcot presenting Blanche to his neurological colleagues, Blanche faints into the outstretched arms of Charcot's assistant Joseph Babinski, with her breasts barely covered, pointing suggestively at Charcot as she turns her head to the side with her face contorted as though in the throes of an orgasm. Remarkably, Wittman remained at the Salpêtrière for 16 years performing as requested for Charcot. Even more remarkable, after release from the hospital, she became a laboratory assistant to Marie Curie and died of radium poisoning.

Hysteria and Hypnosis

Charcot's hysteric rounds really didn't become a hit with the lay public until he began to use hypnosis on his patients. When hypnotized, they would say and do the strangest things. Occasionally, symptoms would transiently disappear or morph into other symptoms. There is a long and convoluted interrelationship between hypnosis and hysteria. Charcot and some others before him believed that only hysterics could be hypnotized. It follows that if we could understand the mechanism of hypnosis, we might develop an insight into the mechanism of hysteria. The origins of hypnosis can be traced to the Austrian physician Franz Anton Mesmer, whose "animal magnetism" was the sensation of Vienna and then Paris in the latter third of the eighteenth century [14].

A major conundrum facing physicians of the time was the mind/body relationship. Traditionally, psychology was a branch of philosophy, a discipline separate from the physical world. However, with the growing realization that diseases of the mind were diseases of the brain, it logically followed that the brain was the anatomical seat of psychic function. There was a growing feeling among many physicians that understanding brain physiology would solve the mind problem, so that psychology might become obsolete. In their daily practices, they frequently saw how psychic events were dependent on the state of brain function. But there were still strong proponents of the dualism theory that the mind and the brain were functionally separate. Mesmer claimed to have discovered a new principle somewhere in between the mind and the brain that allowed him to restore the health of nervous patients. He suggested that nerves communicated between the mind and brain, having features of both. At that time, little was known about how nerves work. Having first experimented with electricity and magnets, Mesmer discovered a power that he considered unique to humans called "animal magnetism." Certain individuals, he in particular, had a special power to influence the brain and cure a wide variety of diseases. He could unleash the mysterious power simply by touching or staring at the patient or by moving his hands over the surface of the body without touching it. He found that he could treat large numbers of patients simultaneously by filling a tub with iron filings, from which protruded rods that the patients could hold onto to receive the stored magnetic energy, a tub full of animal magnetism. Mesmer used background music, sometimes provided by himself with a glass harp, and the great healer, dressed in a lavender silk robe, walked among his thankful patients, touching them with a long, magnetized rod. First in Vienna and then in Paris, members of the established medical community questioned Mesmer's claims, calling him a quack. No doubt the large number of affluent women patients that flocked to Mesmer's séances influenced their thinking. In Paris, a distinguished commission of the Royal Academy that included the well-known French chemist Lavoisier and the American statesman Benjamin Franklin was set up to investigate the claim of quackery. The commission concluded that animal magnetism was a fantasy, a figment of Mesmer's imagination, and that his claims of cure were simply the product of suggestion. Mesmer left Paris and vanished into obscurity, but his animal magnetism remained a fascination in affluent Parisian society and would resurface later as hypnotism.

In the mid-nineteenth century, the Scottish surgeon and "gentleman scientist" James Braid concluded that the trance-like state produced by Mesmer and his followers was due to a physiological state of the brain that he called hypnotism and not due to occult animal magnetism [15]. It was a method of throwing the nervous system into a new condition, something akin to sleep. Braid demonstrated that the process did not require someone with special psychic powers but rather could be done on oneself, autohypnosis. The person simply needed to fix his thoughts, attention and sight on an object and suppress his respiration. He recommended using a small bright object held 18 inches above and in front of the eyes. Clearly, some people were more susceptible to hypnosis than other people. Women were more susceptible than men, but a large segment of the population was susceptible. In one of Baird's exhibitions before 800 people, he was able to hypnotize 10 of 14 men called to the stage to varying degrees. The men focused on a piece of cork attached to their forehead or gazed at objects in the audience. Some of the men remained partially conscious, while others went into a cataleptic-like state with complete insensitivity to pain and no recollection of having been stuck with needles on recovering consciousness. As Baird's observations became widely known, surgeons operated on patients under hypnosis with the patients completely unaware of any pain.

Even more remarkable, subconscious suggestions made during hypnosis could alter subsequent behavior. For example, if one of the men hypnotized by Baird was told to jump up and swing his arms every time he heard the word Christmas, after the hypnotic session was over he would perform the bizarre ritual whenever someone mentioned Christmas, regardless of the appropriateness of the circumstances. Furthermore, he would provide an elaborate explanation for the behavior such as the need to stretch because of a cramp, completely unaware of the real reason for the behavior.

Borderlands of Hypnosis

In America, William A. Hammond, introduced in Chap. 2 as one of the founding fathers of American neurology, noted the similarity of hypnosis with several other altered mental states, including somnambulism (sleep walking), spiritualism and paranormal phenomenon [16]. With each of these conditions, the person appeared to be in a trance-like state with varying degrees of awareness. As with hypnosis, there could be a complete absence of pain, yet people could carry on complex physical activities. After the episode, there was no recollection of the events that took place. Hammond speculated that these mental states represented a type of "automatism" whereby lower brain and spinal cord activity were occurring below the level of conscious awareness. He described one of his patients who developed features of different altered mental states over time. Hammond was asked to see an attractive young lady who was having nightly episodes of somnambulism. She had been under a great deal of emotional stress after the death of her mother and other family members from cholera. Her father had to have a nurse stay with her at night to prevent her from harming herself during one of her sleep-walking episodes. Hammond visited her house late at night to observe an episode. "She was walking very slowly and deliberately, her head elevated, her eyes open, and her hands hanging loosely by her side. We stood aside to let her pass. Without noticing us, she descended the stairs to the parlor, we followed her. Taking a match which she brought with her from her own room, she rubbed it several times on the underside of the mantle-piece until it caught fire, and then turning on the gas, lit it. She next threw herself into an armchair and looked fixedly at a portrait of her mother which hung over the mantle-piece" [17]. Hammond examined her in that position to assess her neurological function. He placed a large book in front of her face blocking her view of the portrait, but she continued to stare in the same direction as though the book wasn't there. He made several threatening movements of his hands as though he was going to strike her in the face, but she made no effort to block the blows. He touched the corners of her eyes with a pencil tip, and she continued to stare without blinking. He then tested her sense of smell and taste, and she did not respond to smelling salts under her nose or pieces of bread soaked in lemon or quinine placed in her half-open mouth. She did not respond to loud noises unexpectedly made next to her ears, scratching her hands with a pin, pulling her hair or pinching her face. Tickling the soles of her feet resulted in withdraw but no laughter or emotion.

After he examined her, she got up from the chair and paced back and forth, wringing her hands and weeping. Hammond took her by the hand and led her back to the chair, where she again sat quietly staring straight ahead. After about 20 minutes he tried to awaken her by first shaking her shoulders and then more violently shaking her head. "She awoke suddenly, looked around her for an instant, as if endeavoring to comprehend her situation, and then burst into a fit of hysterical sobbing. When she recovered her equanimity she had no recollection of anything that had passed, or of having had a dream of any kind" [18].

Hammond noted that the young lady initially improved with "suitable medical treatment" (presumably with bromides, which he commonly used), but then her father notified him that her somnambulism episodes began recurring and, in addition, she was having other spells unrelated to sleep that her father attributed to excessive mental exertion associated with a fanatical interest in philosophy. On revisiting the young lady, Hammond found that she had developed the ability to induce a self-hypnotic state at will. When studying one of her philosophical texts, she would select a section that required intense thought and then fix her gaze straight ahead, not focusing on any particular object and think intensely about what she had just read. This would induce a trance-like state similar to her episodes of somnambulism. "During this state it was said she answered questions correctly, read books held behind her, described scenes passing in distant places, and communicated messages from the dead. She therefore possessed, in every essential aspect, the qualifications of either clairvoyant or a spiritualistic medium, according to the peculiar tenets of belief held by the faithful" [19].

Hammond carefully examined the young woman during one of the episodes of autohypnosis and noted that she was unresponsive to threats and pain, just like during her spells of somnambulism, but she readily responded to questions, making up the answers when necessary. For example, Hammond asked her if there were any spirits in the room, and she answered Socrates, Plato and Schleirmacher (she had just been reading Schleirmacher's Introductions to the Dialogues of Plato). As a ruse, Hammond made up the name of Schleirmacher's constant companion and asked if he was also present. After a brief pause, she reported that his spirit was present and described the man in detail. She was then asked to relay messages from other spirits who came into the room, and she readily reported their dialogue. He then tested her susceptibility to suggestion, telling her she was on a boat at sea in a violent storm and asking if she was frightened. "Yes, I am very much frightened; What shall I do? Oh, save me, save me" [20]. Hammond tested her clairvoyant abilities by asking her questions to which only he knew the answers, and she readily responded with detailed answers, all of them incorrect. He concluded "that she was in a condition similar to that of a dreaming person; for the images and hallucinations were either directly connected with thoughts she had previously had, or were immediately suggested to her through her sense of hearing. Some mental functions were exercised, while others were quiescent. There was no correct judgment and no volition. Imagination, memory, the emotions, and *the ability to be impressed by suggestions,* were present to a high degree" [21]. Hammond described similar phenomena occurring in patients with hysteria, people in the thralls of a religious experience (ecstasy) and clairvoyants conducting a séance. They could be completely insensitive to pain, experience vivid visual illusions and hallucinations, carry on complex physical activities yet have no recollection of the events. Remarkably, he also reported producing similar trance-like states in a wide variety of animals from frogs and snakes to dogs and cats and even lions and a raging bull during which the animals showed no response to pain and became docile. Could such episodes be an inherent feature of the brain?

Nature or Nurture

There is little doubt that Charcot was referring to inherited traits when referring to inherent weakness in patients with hysteria, but relatively little was known about genes and inheritance at the time. Many physicians felt that hysteria was mainly a disease of the affluent upper classes, possibly because the upper classes were the main source of patients in their practice. Charcot argued that inherited susceptibility was not exclusive to any class of society and in fact most of the women at the Salpêtrière with hysteria were from the lower classes [22]. Although others had suggested that men were also susceptible to hysteria, such men were considered effeminate, not "real men." Charcot emphasized that most of the male patients with hysteria that he saw in his out-patient clinic or after 1882 in a special ward that he established at the Salpêtrière were from the laboring class, muscular virile men [23]. Why wouldn't men also inherit susceptibility to hysteria? In people with an inherited diathesis, certain environmental events could precipitate an attack of hysteria. Charcot suggested that traumatic incidents such as industrial and railroad accidents were common precipitating events in men and women. Charcot hinted that ideas and emotions might also be able to precipitate an attack but the notion that psychological trauma might be converted into physical symptoms was not yet in his mindset.

To Charcot, hypnosis was a state of heightened sensitivity to suggestion with a decreased awareness. It is human nature to respond to suggestion but some of us are more responsive to suggestion than others. Why Charcot felt that only patients with hysteria could be hypnotized is not clear. He must have been aware of the many public sessions during which hypnotists (magnetizers) induced a range of symptoms from paralysis to bizarre behaviors in random people from the audience. These public performances were not without skeptics, however; some suggested that the chosen subjects were performing before an audience, while others suggested outright fraud. Similarly, skeptics suggested that Charcot's hysterical patients were cheating both the doctors and audience. Modern views of hypnosis emphasize heightened suggestibility in the setting of a dissociation or disconnection between brain motor control and awareness systems. New functional imaging techniques provide insight into the areas of the brain involved in these processes [24].

Ideas About Hysteria Evolve

In the last years of his career, Charcot began to consider a psychological role in the cause of hysteria [25]. His later experimentation with hypnosis convinced him that ideas could be behind symptoms of hysteria. For example, under hypnosis paralysis could be induced by an idea and, similarly, an idea could cause it to disappear. Yet, the subject was unaware of the idea. Charcot also became particularly interested in the hysterical symptoms that followed psychic trauma, which he called traumatic neurosis. He noted that symptoms produced by hypnosis could be identical to symptoms produced by psychic trauma. Both resulted from an idea; with hypnosis the idea came from the suggestion of the hypnotizer, and with traumatic neurosis from auto-suggestion. When he hypnotized patients with traumatic neurosis, he could reproduce the symptoms by reenacting the original psychic trauma, similar to the observations by Breuer and Freud in Vienna (see Chap. 4). In the last few years of his life, Charcot moved even further toward a psychological explanation for hysteria when he appointed a young psychologist, Pierre Janet, to lead an experimental psychology laboratory in the Salpêtrière. In his work with Charcot, Janet concluded that emotional trauma in one's past could cause symptoms of hysteria, which, like hypnotic suggestions, were a type of dissociated consciousness. He was the first to introduce the concept of dissociation to explain hysteria. In an article published in the last year of his life, Charcot marveled at the remarkable influence of the mind and ideas on the body, particularly in susceptible individuals. But even with that he emphasized that there is no idea without modification on nerve signals in some region of the brain. In other words, the mind is the brain.

Remarkably, Charcot's "la grande hystérie" largely disappeared within a decade of his death [26]. Charcot's loyal disciple Joseph Babinski, famous in neurology circles for his great toe sign, later noted that during Charcot's time not a day went by without a patient having an hysterical crisis, and often many patients were seized simultaneously or successively. Within a few years of his death, such seizures virtually disappeared. Jules-Joseph Dejerine, who took over for Charcot a few years after his death, laid down the law to patients and staff alike that hysterical crises would not be tolerated. He was brutal with hysterical patients, and he later boasted that during his 8 years at the Salpêtrière he rarely saw a hysterical fit. Babinski, being a Charcot protégé, took longer to distance himself from the great master's thinking on hysteria but eventually developed his own ideas on hysteria. It was simply a symptom that could be induced by suggestion and abolished by persuasion, and it could be transitory and not necessarily inborn or a life-long disability. Another famous former pupil of Charcot, Georges Gilles de la Tourette (of Tourette syndrome), distanced himself from Charcot's fascination with the ovaries in hysteria and warned against ovarian surgery as a treatment.

If there is one lesson we can learn from Charcot and his "la grande hystérie," it's that physicians play an important role in molding symptoms in patients with psychogenic illness. After Charcot, fits no longer were in vogue, but sensory symptoms such as headache, dizziness, generalized body pain and fatigue continued to occur in the same patient population. There was a shift from dramatic motor symptoms to more subtle sensory symptoms. Via suggestion, physicians play a critical role in determining which sensory symptoms will be experienced and how long they last. I have personally observed how symptoms in patients with psychogenic illness change and multiply as they are referred from one specialist to another. Like a blind man, each subspecialist "feels" the elephant from their particular perspective, focusing on symptoms in their particular area and often missing the overall picture.

Neurasthenia and Neurosis

Tainted by Charcot's "circus," a century of sadistic treatments and a changing symptom complex, the diagnosis of hysteria began to lose its luster in the late nineteenth century. Furthermore, many physicians felt uneasy in making a diagnosis of hysteria in their male patients. Diagnoses such as spleen and hypochondriasis had been used for men with hysterical symptoms, but these terms were rooted in archaic concepts that no longer seemed relevant. In Germany the term nervosity (nervosität) and in England and America the term neurasthenia became popular for describing a wide range of physical and mental symptoms seen in men and women and felt to be of "nervous" origin. Neurasthenia, a general physical and mental exhaustion, had been part of the hysteria symptom complex dating back to ancient times. But neurasthenia was redefined in 1869, when an American electrotherapist in New York, George Beard, published an article describing neurasthenia as a functional nervous disorder with a wide range of symptoms [27]. He claimed that he had successfully treated a number of such patients with electrotherapy. In 1880, Beard's book, *American Nervousness,* established neurasthenia as the most common nervous disorder in men and women [28]. Symptoms ranged from fatigue, headache, body pain and insomnia to numbness and paralysis. He concluded that the symptoms were due to lack of "nervous force" resulting from subtle chemical changes in the brain. Beard's neurasthenia rapidly took hold in America and Europe, where it became a fashionable diagnosis of the rapidly expanding affluent middle classes.

Beard saw neurasthenia from a unique American perspective. He felt that the American drive to be successful and the pace of modern life provoked nervous disorders. Beard noted that scientific discoveries such as the telegraph and steam engine increased the pace of daily life and this, along with the constant drive to get ahead, overtaxed the nervous system and led to a breakdown. Furthermore, Beard pointed out that neurasthenia was a disease of high achievers, those who were most exposed to the stresses of modern living. Thus, neurasthenia became a status diagnosis, and even Beard considered himself among the affected. Sigmund Freud and many prominent European intellectuals also considered themselves neurasthenics. Although initially neurasthenia was diagnosed more often in men than in women, it really wasn't the male version of hysteria since it was rapidly replacing the diagnosis of hysteria in both men and women. Beard felt strongly that neurasthenia was a real physical illness and not a sign of a weak will or malingering.

Americanitis

Around the same time, the term Americanitis became popular in the lay press [29]. The exact origin of the term is unclear, but the American psychologist William James (brother of writer Henry James) is credited with popularizing its use. Stated simply, Americanitis was Beard's neurasthenia. The hustle and bustle of routine American life caused a unique nervous disorder with a range of symptoms. Americans were nervous because they were driven to get ahead and acquire material gains, but often their goals were unattainable. The suggested cure for Americanitis in men was to stop worrying and be happy with what they had. Work less and play tag with their children. Women should use the family meal to reform their husband and children by forcing them to eat slowly and carefully chew their food. By the early twentieth century, just about every physical or social ill in America was being blamed on Americanitis. The ultimate "cure" for Americanitis was the Great Depression in 1929; by the mid-1930s the term was largely forgotten.

As in Europe, neurology in America was a newly developing subspecialty in the latter part of the nineteenth century. It became generally accepted that all human behavior was mediated by electrical signals moving through nerves in the brain, so it followed that modifying the electrical signals could modify abnormal behavior. The mind and the brain were one and the same. Neurologists assured their patients that they were the ones to treat their nervous prostration, headaches, dizziness, insomnia and emotional irritability. They had a range of drugs at their disposal, including sedatives such as chloral hydrate, bromides, and opioids and stimulants such as caffeine and cocaine. Electrotherapy in its various forms was used to "shake up" the nervous system, and dramatic cures for hysteria and neurasthenia were claimed [30]. As with their European colleagues, there were some who wondered whether their patients' symptoms were real or just imaginary. All had to admit, however, that their symptoms, whether real or fake, were tenaciously held, often at the cost of considerable personal and social loss. The young American neurologist Silas Weir Mitchell agreed with his New York colleague George Beard that hysteria and neurasthenia were real nervous disorders and not imagined symptoms. In many ways, Mitchell was the Charcot of American neurology.

Silas Weir Mitchell and the Civil War

Weir Mitchell (he preferred Weir) was born in 1829, the son of a prominent Philadelphia doctor [31]. He graduated from the Jefferson Medical College at age 21 in 1850 and traveled through Europe for a year, spending a brief time in Paris with the famous physiologist, Claude Bernard. Mitchell was fond of quoting Bernard's response to his naive speculations, "Why think when you can experiment?" "Exhaust experiment and then think," said Bernard [32]. When Mitchell returned to the United States, he joined his father's busy clinical practice and began a research program on snake venoms. In the process, he developed a life-long close relationship with William Hammond, who, as mentioned earlier, was the Surgeon General of the United States during the Civil War. He and Hammond were about the same age, had productive medical and literary careers, and both went on to become prominent leaders in American neurology. Together they published two papers on snake venoms in 1859. He later compared his experience working on science and fiction and emphasized the importance of maintaining an open mind with both endeavors. "Above all, when engaged in any form of production, my mind is turned on to it as one winds a piece of machinery and waits to see it grind out results. I seem to be dealing with ideas which come from what I call my mind but as to the mechanism of this process, beyond a certain point it is absolutely mystery. I say, 'I will think this over. How does it look? To what does it lead?' Then there comes to me from some inward somewhere criticisms, suggestions, in a word, ideas, about the ultimate origin of which I know nothing" [33].

With the onset of the American Civil war, Mitchell accepted a position as a contract surgeon for the Union Army. Although he arranged a commission for his brother, Mitchell did not join the Union Army himself. His father became ill and had to give up his practice in 1855. After his father's death and Mitchell's marriage in 1859, Mitchell was the sole provider for an extended family, and he chose to pay someone else to take his place in the army. This decision haunted Mitchell throughout his life, and he often wondered what it would be like to fight in a military battle. In his novels, he relied on anecdotes from friends and patients who took part in the major battles of the Civil War. Mitchell was first stationed at the old armory building on 16th Street that was serving as a Union Hospital. It was here that Mitchell first became interested in nervous disorders, and he convinced Surgeon General Hammond to devote a large ward solely to the treatment of such disorders [34]. Mitchell's initial impression of neurasthenia was that little was known about the cause and treatments were largely ineffective. He did favor milder treatments such as rest, massage and a healthy diet, but he was also a proponent of electrotherapy. As the number of wounded soldiers exponentially increased, Mitchell was moved to a much larger hospital at Turner's Lane, called the "Stump Hospital" by the soldiers. Here, Mitchell, along with colleagues George Reed Morehouse and William Williams Keen, focused on nerve injuries. Mitchell, who coined the term phantom limb, noted that 95% of men experienced some feeling of the limb still being present after amputation. Most reported that the phantom limb felt shorter than the real limb, and most complained of pain in the phantom limb. Mitchell, along with colleagues Morehouse and Keen, published a classic textbook on pain and wartime injuries in 1864 [35]. The book provided detailed descriptions of the wide range of painful conditions associated with gunshot injuries. The most dramatic pain syndrome described in the book would later become known as causalgia, combining the Greek words for heat and pain. The soldiers described the pain as "burning," "mustard red hot" or like a "red hot file rasping the skin." It most commonly involved the palms of the hands or the back of the feet. Mitchell and colleagues noted that the pain made the sufferer anxious and irritable and markedly interfered with sleep. They tried a range of treatments including counterirritants and injecting morphine into the painful site all with little benefit. Many of the soldiers begged to have the painful limb amputated. Mitchell and his colleagues described the case of a seventeen-year-old Pennsylvania boy who was shot in the shoulder at the Battle of Gettysburg. After recovering from the acute injury, he began suffering from a severe burning pain in his hand that made him "nervous and hysterical." The only thing that brought him relief was to wear loose cotton gloves on both hands that he kept wet by regularly sprinkling water onto them. The young soldier became so despondent that his family was worried he was going insane.

The Rest Cure

After the war, Mitchell returned to a lucrative neurological private practice in Philadelphia that was largely funded by affluent women suffering from hysteria and neurasthenia. Based on his experience with soldiers during the Civil War and patients in his private practice, he developed the so-called "rest cure" that received worldwide notoriety [36]. In a conversation with his close friend and fellow physician William Osler, Mitchell suggested that a woman patient provided the initial inspiration for the rest cure [37]. The highly intelligent woman completed her degree at a prominent Boston college in 3 years and then married and had four children in rapid sequence. This was followed by a complete mental breakdown with extreme fatigue and a diagnosis of nervous exhaustion or neurasthenia. Doctors recommended exercise, but she refused to get out of bed. When Mitchell saw her, she was pale and thin and was eating relatively little. He decided to let her stay in bed and increase her food intake. Remarkably, she had a complete recovery, returning to her wifely duties, including having several more children. Paradoxically, despite his promotion of the rest cure, Mitchell repeatedly emphasized the importance of exercise for good mental health, particularly for his women patients with neurasthenia. In fact, he suggested that one potential benefit of the rest cure was that it made women eager to return to normal activities, including exercise. Anecdotes indicated that Mitchell would resort to extreme methods to force his women patients out of bed to exercise [38]. On one occasion, he drove a patient halfway home, where he left her to walk the rest of the way on her own, and on another, he threatened to disrobe and get into bed with the patient if she did not get up. Although the latter anecdote seems out of character considering Mitchell's prudish outlook regarding sex, it was reported by multiple sources.

Mitchell believed that both men and women were susceptible to hysteria and neurasthenia but women were particularly susceptible because of their weak constitution. He felt that young girls between the ages of 14 and 18 were at particular risk and that it was probably best not to try to educate girls in that age range. Their limited energy was best directed towards developing skills required for their future roles as wives and mothers rather than being wasted on mental pursuits. Mitchell wrote not only medical books for academics but also for the lay public. His best-selling book on nervous disorders, *Wear and Tear, or Hints for the Overworked,* summarizes his misogynistic views on women's mental health [39]. Young women whose nervous systems were overtaxed with misguided mental pursuits were destined to "the shawl and the sofa, neuralgia, weak backs, and the varied forms of hysteria, that domestic demon which has produced untold discomfort in many households...only the doctor knows what one of these self-made invalids can do to make a household wretched" [40]. He outlined his rest cure for nervous disorders in another medical advice book, *Fat and Blood: An Essay on the Treatment of Current Forms of Neurasthenia and Hysteria* [41]. The wear and tear that women were so susceptible to required an extended period of bed rest with forced-feeding. Mitchell noted that men with neurasthenia didn't do so well with his rest cure, so for these patients, which included Walt Whitman, he recommended the "West cure." Patients were instructed to visit the West to engage in vigorous physical activity and to write about their experiences [42]. Owen Wister Jr., the son of Mitchell's cousin and life-long friend Sarah Butler Wister, wrote the cowboy novel *The Virginian* during his travels in the West, which were prescribed by Mitchell in 1884 for his bout of neur-asthenia [43]. Mitchell recommended yearly vacations for both men and women to break the build-up in stress from work and household duties.

Mitchell's rest cure for women was much more than just a nice rest [44]. The women were sequestered from their family to prevent interference and were con-fined to bed for 6 to 8 weeks. At least initially they had to move their bowels and pass urine while lying in bed. Twice a day in the morning and evening, they were lifted onto a bedside lounge where they stayed while their bed was remade. Throughout the day, they were constantly fed great amounts of high-fat foods, including up to two gallons of milk. This was done to restore the "fat and blood" that was presumably depleted by stress and overwork. The cruelest part of the treat-ment was that they were prohibited from reading, writing or performing any type of intellectual activity. Not even manual tasks such as sewing or crocheting were per-mitted. In place of physical activity, they received massages and electrical stimula-tion of their muscles. In addition to "restoration of fat and blood," success of the rest cure depended on a common-sense psychotherapy provided by Mitchell. The pro-cess included "the firm kindness of a well-trained nurse" [45]. Mitchell was well aware that the physician was a powerful force in determining the success of any type of treatment. In his book *Fat and Blood,* Mitchell wrote, "If the physician has the force of character required to secure the confidence and respect of his patients he has also much more in his power, and should have the tact to seize the proper occa-sion to direct the thoughts of his patients to the lapse from duties to others, and to the selfishness which a life of invalidism is apt to bring about" [46]. He also recog-nized that some physicians had the power to help the healing process, while others did not: "Mere hygienic advice will win a victory in the hands of one man and obtain no good results in those of another, for we are, after all, artists who all use the same means to an end but fail or succeed according to our method of using them" [47].

Mitchell's rest cure rapidly became popular in Europe and America, particularly for young women with eating disorders, anorexia hysteria or anorexia nervosa. Charcot apparently was so impressed with the results of the treatment that late in his career, he began to consider the possibility that hysteria was a psychogenic illness rather than a neurological disease. But how did the women who underwent Mitchell's rest cure feel about it? Most took their medicine meekly, giving the great nerve doc-tor his due for his wonderful cure. Likely a rest away from the stress of wifely and family responsibilities was helpful for their mental health. The fact that many nearly doubled their weight during the cure couldn't have done much for their self-esteem, however. Among Mitchell's patients were several prominent socialites and novel-ists, Charlotte Perkins Gilman, Winifred Howells, Edith Wharton, and Virginia Woolf. Mitchell nearly drove Gilman mad with his advice to drop all of her creative writing endeavors. Gilman, who was in a failed marriage and probably suffered from postpartum depression, later wrote "using the remnants of intelligence that remained, and helped by a wise friend, I cast the noted specialist's advice to the winds and went to work again--work, the normal life of every human being; work, in which is joy and growth and service, without which one is a pauper and a parasite--ultimately recovering some measure of power" [48]. Gilman achieved a modicum of revenge when she later published a short story *The Yellow Wallpaper* in 1892, describing in the first person, a young woman's plunge toward insanity when she was forced to avoid all physical and mental activity with the rest cure [49]. Many psychiatrists (called alienists at the time) lauded the story as one of the best descriptions of mental illness ever written. Other physicians warned patients against reading the story because it might drive them insane. Gilman responded that her goal was not to frighten women but to save them from the terrible experience that she had undergone with the rest cure. This is somewhat surprising since Gilman initially described the rest cure as "agreeable" [50]. After being sent a copy, Mitchell called *The Yellow Wallpaper* "blood curdling" [51] and later hinted that it influenced his thinking about the rest cure. The story of Winifred Howells is even more tragic [52]. After 8 years of suffering from a chronic illness diagnosed as hysteria, Winifred's parents, who lived in New York, decided to send her to Mitchell for his rest cure. At age 25 she weighed only 57 pounds. This was a difficult decision for the parents since the cost of the treatment program was about $2000 or about $50,000 in today's currency. Winifred did gain about 10 pounds with the forced feeding, but her symptoms continued to progress and after a few months in Pennsylvania she died suddenly of heart failure. Autopsy confirmed that she had an organic disease, not hysteria.

Many saw Mitchell's rest cure as a compassionate, effective treatment for hysteria and neurasthenia. At the time, there weren't a lot of other treatment options available. Regardless of one's opinion of the effectiveness of Mitchell's rest cure, it did make Mitchell a wealthy man. The demand for the treatment was so great that Mitchell developed a series of satellite rest treatment centers in and around Philadelphia run by women nurses he personally trained. At its peak, Mitchell's medical practice was one of the largest in the United States, with a yearly income of more than $100,000, or $2,500,000 in today's currency [53].

Silas Weir Mitchell, the Enigma

As an American neurologist, I can't help but have mixed feelings regarding Weir Mitchell. He made significant contributions to the burgeoning field of neurology, particularly his work on snake venoms and nerve injuries, and he, along with Hammond, was one of the founding fathers of American neurology. He was elected the first president of the American Neurological Association and later to the National Academy of Sciences. But his legacy is tainted by his paternalistic and misogynistic views, which were not uncommon in male physicians of the time. Like Charlotte Perkins Gilman, some women patients saw Mitchell as vain and aloof with little empathy, but others, such as the Chicago writer and feminist Amelia Gere Mason, with whom Mitchell maintained a life-long correspondence, saw him as a caring physician and friend [54]. Although Mason and several other women intellectuals who regularly corresponded with Mitchell disagreed with his views on women's role in society, they found him to be a caring physician who was open to listening to opposing arguments, but steadfastly maintained his antifeminist opinions. In 1895, Dean Agnes Irwin invited Mitchell to speak to the young ladies in the first class of Radcliffe College. Mitchell provided helpful suggestions about the importance of exercise and outdoor activities to balance their studies, but he also made clear his opposition to women entering professional careers. In a remarkable display of hubris, he closed the speech with, "I see the wrecks come ashore to sail the seas of success no more. Is it any wonder I wish to warn those who are sailing or about to sail on treacherous seas? I hope, my dear Dean, and you, ladies, that no wreck from these shores will be drifted into my dockyard. Sometimes I can refit the ruined craft. Alas! Sometimes I cannot" [55].

None can doubt that Mitchell had a creative mind and was a prolific writer. In addition to more than a hundred scientific articles and books, he published more than 50 literary titles including novels, essays and poems. In his later years, he regularly produced one or two novels a year up to the age of 83 and was a leading-selling American author of fiction at the turn of the century. I inherited several of his novels when our departmental library did some housecleaning, and although they would not be considered great literature they were entertaining and provided insight into his thinking process. His strength was in character development, particularly women characters, many of which had features of neurasthenia. In *Constance Trescot,* published in 1905 when he was 76 years old, Mitchell created a strong-willed woman who would stop at nothing to avenge the murder of her husband [56]. Constance was "one of those rare women who for good or ill, attract because of some inexplicable quality of sex. Incapable of analysis, it accounts for divorces and ruined households, even for suicides or murders" [57]. His best-selling book *Hugh Wynne,* published in 1896, was a historical saga of the Revolutionary War told by Hugh in the first person but also at times in the third person by intertwining a diary of his friend [58]. Hugh Wynne's description of his Philadelphia family's "Quaker habit of absolute self-repression, and of concealment of emotion" [59] no doubt reflected aspects of Mitchell's own upbringing in Philadelphia a century later. The book sold over 500,000 copies. Mitchell boasted that he never wrote a line in any of his novels that might cause a young girl to blush. According to Mitchell's biographer, Ernest Earnest, " Few intellectual leaders have achieved greatness without first seeing through the shame and stupidities of their times. Mitchell was a great man in his era; he did not transcend it" [60]. Somehow his fiction always got bogged down in "Victorian muck."

Probably Mitchell's most important legacy was his approach to patients with psychosomatic symptoms. He used a combination of insight and pragmatism along with a strong belief that patients could be helped. Mitchell was not wed to a specific scientific theory, but he did understand the importance of the interrelationship between the mind and the body in generating symptoms. He used common sense in treating symptoms, whatever it took. On one occasion, Mitchell prescribed daily champagne and a lady's maid for a young, wealthy New England woman after curing her neurasthenia with his rest cure. The woman's prohibitionist mother later wrote Mitchell to condemn the prescription, noting "her daughter might be purchasing bodily comfort and ease, health and enjoyment at the cost of her immortal soul" [61]. On the other hand, Mitchell wasn't above threatening his young lady patients with a whipping if they refused to follow his instructions. Mitchell recognized that symptoms often had a deeper meaning than appeared at the surface, and it was important to provide patients with insight into their condition. He had little use for psychoanalysis and found Freud's sexual theories repulsive. Above all else, Mitchell was self-assured and confident in his abilities, and always provided his patients with positive reassurance. He believed that medicine was an art, and he had a unique ability to communicate medical ideas to his patients, a trait rare among medical professionals. He spent much of his life writing and reading books, devouring two or three novels a week. His love for books is apparent in his poem *Books and the Man,* written in 1898. In a eulogy after Mitchell's death in 1914, his war-time colleague William Keen called him "yeasty man" because of his fertile mind.

> "Of the proud peerage of the mind are they,
> Fair, courteous gentlemen who wait our will.
> When come the lonely hours the scholar loves,
> And glows the hearth and all the house is still." [62].

Nerve Doctors

By the last few decades of the nineteenth century, the reflex theory of nervous diseases, with its gynecological focus, was largely abandoned throughout Europe. More and more gynecologists considered the theory ridiculous and warned against needless gynecological procedures that often only aggravated the problem. William Playfair, a leading London gynecologist who was one of the first to introduce Mitchell's rest cure in Europe, strongly discouraged procedures on the pelvic organs for treating neurosis [63]. He emphasized that the last thing a nervous, anxious woman needed was to have repeated vaginal examinations and undergo procedures to correct a slight displacement of the uterus, cauterize the cervix or scrape out the uterine lining. These procedures had their place for treating gynecological diseases but not for treating nervous disorders. Besides, men and children could have the same nervous symptoms as women but were not susceptible to gynecological diseases.

The newly developing specialty of psychiatry began to compete for the care of the potentially large population of affluent women and men with neurotic symptoms. Overall, this new breed of "nerve doctors" focused on the central nervous system as the seat of the problem and also ridiculed physicians who still focused on spinal reflex theory and the female genitourinary system. Wilhelm Griesinger, a leading German psychiatrist in the late nineteenth century, felt that psychiatric and neurologic diseases were the same, both brain diseases [64]. Griesinger borrowed the notion of excessive brain excitability from Romberg and suggested that the more excited the brain became the more likely one would develop neurosis. An irritated and excited brain could not function efficiently, analogous to a motor running out of gear. Like Charcot, he also felt that there was an inherited susceptibility to neurosis, so that certain people were more susceptible to "irritable weakness." At the University of Vienna, the leading academic psychiatrist Theodor Meynert studied postmortem brains in search of the pathology of mental illness and suggested that psychiatric diseases were diseases of the forebrain. At that time in Vienna, psychiatrists were called neuropathologists because of their focus on brain pathology. While many, like Charcot, thought that pathology would eventually be found for all psychiatric illnesses, others distinguished between psychosis and neurosis, with the former being an organic brain disease and the latter a milder functional disorder of the nervous system without demonstrable pathology.

Evolution and the Brain

The publication of Charles Darwin's *On the Origin of Species* in 1859 hit the scientific world like a thunderbolt, and within 20 years his theory of evolution was largely accepted as fact. It impacted all areas of science but probably none more than neuroscience. As one moves out the evolutionary tree, more complex brain structures evolve with higher and higher levels of complexity. Lower-level reflexive behavior remains, but under the control of the higher centers. For example, in humans, reflex withdraw of an extremity from a painful stimulus occurs through nerve connections in the spinal cord, although these "automatic" reflexes are modulated by higher brain levels. Primitive reactions such as body postures, grimacing and "knitting" of the brow are "reflex"-like behaviors ingrained in primitive levels of the evolving brain. In his book *The Expression of Emotions in Man and Animals* (1872), Darwin [65] suggested that these types of facial expressions were generated by predetermined nerve cell connections like a "habit." He kept a daily log on the development of his own son and concluded that expressions such as crying and frowning were reflex actions reinforced by habit and did not imply awareness. Although these reflex facial expressions were "hard wired" in the primitive brain, he felt that a certain amount of practice was needed for full expression.

The concept of an evolutionary primitive "emotional brain" underlying a more advanced "thinking brain" dates back to the late nineteenth century and the famous English neurologist John Hughlings Jackson. Jackson, who was greatly influenced by Darwin, felt that evolution of the brain involved the build-up of increasingly complex structures on top of more primitive structures. Jackson theorized that diseases like psychosis and dementia occurred when lower primitive centers were released from higher cortical centers. Such a release from higher cortical control could make the most civilized man act like his primitive ancestors, a kind of reverse evolution. Jackson, who was apprenticed to local physicians in York, England at the age of 15, had no formal university training but would go on to have a great influence on the developing field of neurology. He is probably best known for his description of the slow march of muscle jerking along an extremity during a focal motor epileptic seizure, a "Jacksonian seizure." From this observation, he surmised that there must be a topographical localization of different parts of the body on the motor cortex in the frontal lobe. Sigmund Freud was strongly influenced by Jackson. Freud's id was the primitive brain with raw passions and drives, and his ego was the cognitive brain that prevented these passions and drives from breaking into consciousness.

Hughling Jackson's evolutionary model` of brain development could explain psychogenic motor phenomena with hysteria such as paralysis and fits, since more primitive emotional and reflex centers deep in the brain were under the control of evolutionarily advanced cortical centers. With chronic threat to life and limb, emotions such as fear gain the upper hand over cognitive faculties and primitive behaviors like paralysis and fits occur. The concept of discreet brain centers for different functions was evolving, and neurologists were aware that patients could have dissociations between function and awareness. For example, some patients with paralysis due to a stroke deny the paralysis and make up a story to explain why they can't move their arm when asked to. The idea of localized brain damage causing symptoms due to disconnection of one brain center from another was just taking shape. A small stroke in the back of the brain on the left side can disconnect the visual and speech centers so that the patient cannot name an object they are presented, yet they are perfectly aware of how to use it. It was not so farfetched to imagine a situation where cognitive centers could be unaware of activity originating in more primitive emotional centers. As we will see in the next chapter, Sigmund Freud used the evolutionary model of brain organization to construct a psychological model of the mind to explain normal and abnormal human behavior.

In Brief

The nineteenth century saw a gradual evolution in the clinical profile of hysteria from predominantly motor symptoms such as paralysis and fits to sensory symptoms such as headache, backache, fatigue and dizziness. By the end of the century, the classical picture of hysteria was rarely seen and the diagnosis of hysteria was largely replaced with more socially acceptable diagnoses such as neurosis and neurasthenia. In America, symptoms of neurasthenia were attributed to a stressful lifestyle, and treatments focused on rest and avoidance of stress. It wasn't until the twentieth century, however, that the link between chronic stress and psychosomatic symptoms became firmly established.

References

1. Porter R. The body and the mind, the doctor and the patient: negotiating hysteria. In: Gilman SL, King H, Porter R, et al., editors. Hysteria beyond Freud. Berkeley: University California Press; 1993. p. 242.
2. Briquet P. Traité de l'Hystérie. Paris: JB Bailiére et Fils; 1859.
3. Briquet P. Traité de l'Hystérie, vol. 1859. Paris: JB Bailiére et Fils. p. 3.

4. Mai FM, Merskey H. Briquet's treatise on hysteria. A synopsia and commentary. Arch Gen Psychiatry. 1980;37:1401–5.
5. Briquet P. Traité de l'Hystérie, vol. 1859. Paris: JB Bailiére et Fils. p. 47.
6. Briquet P. Traité de l'Hystérie, vol. 1859. Paris: JB Bailiére et Fils. p. 584.
7. Briquet P. Traité de l'Hystérie, vol. 1859. Paris: JB Bailiére et Fils. p. 98–9.
8. Briquet P. Traité de l'Hystérie, vol. 1859. Paris: JB Bailiére et Fils. p. 115.
9. Briquet P. Traité de l'Hystérie, vol. 1859. Paris: JB Bailiére et Fils. p. 207.
10. Briquet P. Traité de l'Hystérie, vol. 1859. Paris: JB Bailiére et Fils. p. 371.
11. Shorter E. From paralysis to fatigue: a history of psychosomatic illness in the modern era. New York: Free Press; 1992. p. 166–200.
12. Scull A. Hysteria: the disturbing history. New York: Oxford University Press; 2009. p. 111.
13. Charcot JM. Lectures on the diseases of the nervous system, iii, vol. 1889. London: New Sydenham Society. p. 13–8.
14. Ellenberger H. The discovery of the unconscious. New York: Basic Books; 1970.
15. Braid J. Neurypnology. London: Churchill; 1843.
16. Hammond WA. On certain conditions of nervous derangement, somnambulism – hypnosis – hysteria – Hysteroid affections, ETC. New York: G.P. Putnam's Sons; 1881.
17. Hammond WA. On certain conditions of nervous derangement, somnambulism – hypnosis – hysteria – Hysteroid affections, ETC, vol. 1881. New York: G.P. Putnam's Sons. p. 3.
18. Hammond WA. On certain conditions of nervous derangement, somnambulism – hypnosis – hysteria – Hysteroid affections, ETC, vol. 1881. New York: G.P. Putnam's Sons. p. 5.
19. Hammond WA. On certain conditions of nervous derangement, somnambulism – hypnosis – hysteria – Hysteroid affections, ETC, vol. 1881. New York: G.P. Putnam's Sons. p. 10.
20. Hammond WA. On certain conditions of nervous derangement, somnambulism – hypnosis – hysteria – Hysteroid affections, ETC, vol. 1881. New York: G.P. Putnam's Sons. p. 14.
21. Hammond WA. On certain conditions of nervous derangement, somnambulism – hypnosis – hysteria – Hysteroid affections, ETC, vol. 1881. New York: G.P. Putnam's Sons. p. 15.
22. Scull A. Hysteria: the disturbing history. New York: Oxford University Press; 2009. p. 125–7.
23. Micale MS. Charcot and the idea of hysteria in the male: gender, mental science, and medical diagnosis in late nineteenth-century France. Med Hist. 1990;34:363–411.
24. Hoeft F, Gabrieli JDE, Whitfield-Gabrieli S, Haas BW, Bammer R, Menon V, et al. Functional brain basis of hypnotizability. Arch Gen Psychiatry. 2012;69:1064–72.
25. Shorter E. From paralysis to fatigue: a history of psychosomatic illness in the modern era. New York: Free Press; 1992. p. 193–6.
26. Shorter E. From paralysis to fatigue: a history of psychosomatic illness in the modern era. New York: Free Press; 1992. p. 196–200.
27. Beard G. Neurasthenia or nervous exhaustion. Br Med Stud J. 1869;80:217–21.
28. Beard G. American nervousness. New York: Putnam; 1881.
29. Beck J. 'Americanitis': The disease of living too fast. The Atlantic, 2016 March 11.
30. Gilman SL. Electrotherapy and mental illness: then and now. Hist Psychiatry. 2008;19:339–57.
31. Earnest E. S. Weir Mitchell, novelist and physician. Philadelphia: University of Pennsylvania Press; 1950.
32. Earnest E. S. Weir Mitchell, novelist and physician. Philadelphia: University of Pennsylvania Press; 1950. p. 26.
33. Burr AR. Weir Mitchell, his life and letters. New York: Duffield and Co; 1929. p. 76–7.
34. Mitchell SW. Some personal recollections of the Civil war. Philadelphia: Transactions of the College of Physicians of Philadelphia; 1905.
35. Mitchell SW, Morehouse GR, Keen WW. Gunshot wounds and other injuries of nerves. Philadelphia: Lippincott and Co.; 1864.
36. Mitchell SW. Rest in nervous disease: its use and abuse. In: Seguin EG, editor. A series of American clinical lectures, Vol. 1, no. 4. New York: Putnam; 1875.
37. Earnest E. S. Weir Mitchell, novelist and physician. Philadelphia: University of Pennsylvania Press; 1950. p. 81.

38. Earnest E. S. Weir Mitchell, novelist and physician. Philadelphia: University of Pennsylvania Press; 1950. p. 83.
39. Mitchell SW. Wear and tear or hints for the over worked. 5th ed. Philadelphia: Lippincott; 1891.
40. Mitchell SW. Wear and tear or hints for the over worked. 5th ed. Philadelphia: Lippincott; 1891. p. 32.
41. Mitchell SW. Fat and blood: an essay on the treatment of certain forms of neurasthenia and hysteria. Philadelphia: Lippincott; 1889.
42. Stiles A. Go rest, young man. Monitor Psychol. 2012;43:32.
43. Schuster DG. Personalizing illness and modernity: S Weir Mitchell, literary women, and neurasthenia, 1870-1914. Bull Hist Med. 2005;712
44. Mitchell SW. Fat and blood: an essay on the treatment of certain forms of neurasthenia and hysteria. Philadelphia: Lippincott; 1889. p. 51.
45. Earnest E. S. Weir Mitchell, novelist and physician. Philadelphia: University of Pennsylvania Press; 1950. p. 83.
46. Earnest E. S. Weir Mitchell, novelist and physician. Philadelphia: University of Pennsylvania Press; 1950. p. 84.
47. Earnest E. S. Weir Mitchell, novelist and physician. Philadelphia: University of Pennsylvania Press; 1950. p. 85.
48. Gilman CP. Why I wrote the Yellow Wallpaper. The Forerunner, October, 1913.
49. Stetson CP. The Yellow Wall-paper. A story. The New England Magazine. 1892;11:647–56.
50. Cervetti N. S Weir Mitchell, 1829–1914. Philadelphia's literary physician. University Park, PA: Penn State University Press; 2012. p. 148.
51. Cervetti N. S Weir Mitchell, 1829–1914. Philadelphia's literary physician. University Park, PA: Penn State University Press; 2012. p. 150.
52. Cervetti N. S Weir Mitchell, 1829–1914. Philadelphia's literary physician. University Park, PA: Penn State University Press; 2012. p. 143–4.
53. Tucker BR. S. Weir Mitchell: a brief sketch of his life with personal recollections. Boston: Richard G. Badger; 1914. p. 15.
54. Schuster DG. Personalizing illness and modernity: S Weir Mitchell, literary women, and neurasthenia, 1870–1914. Bull Hist Med. 2005:703–11.
55. Cervetti N. S Weir Mitchell, 1829–1914. Philadelphia's literary physician. University Park, PA: Penn State University Press; 2012. p. 187.
56. Mitchell SW. Constance Trescot. New York: The Century Co; 1905.
57. Earnest ES. Weir Mitchell, novelist and physician. Philadelphia: University of Pennsylvania Press; 1950. p. 185.
58. Mitchell SW. Hugh Wynne. Free Quaker: sometime brevet lieutenant-colonel on the staff of his excellency General Washington. New York: The Century Co; 1904.
59. Mitchell SW. Hugh Wynne. Free Quaker: sometime brevet lieutenant-colonel on the staff of his excellency General Washington. New York: The Century Co; 1904. p. 131.
60. Earnest ES. Weir Mitchell, novelist and physician. Philadelphia: University of Pennsylvania Press; 1950. p. 236.
61. Earnest ES. Weir Mitchell, novelist and physician. Philadelphia: University of Pennsylvania Press; 1950. p. 228.
62. Mitchell SW. Complete poems of S. Weir Mitchell. New York: The Century Co; 1914.
63. Shorter E. From paralysis to fatigue: a history of psychosomatic illness in the modern era. New York: Free Press; 1992. p. 206.
64. Shorter E. From paralysis to fatigue: a history of psychosomatic illness in the modern era. New York: Free Press; 1992. p. 208–10.
65. Darwin C. The expression of the emotions in man and animals. London: John Murray; 1872.

Psychosomatic Illness in the Twentieth Century

4

> *Just as scientists prematurely proclaimed infectious disease to be dead, so too psychiatrists prematurely announced the death of hysteria.*
>
> Elaine Showalter. [1]

By the end of the nineteenth century, the diagnosis of neurasthenia was one of the most common medical diagnoses in Europe and America. But the diagnosis had alternate meanings to different people. To the average layperson, it meant a kind of generalized nervousness, a case of "the nerves." To some psychiatrists, it was considered the same as neurosis or psychoneurosis, a mild functional disorder of the nervous system with physical symptoms to be distinguished from more severe nervous system disorders such as dementia and psychosis. Others used the term as the equivalent of hysteria. Both were considered to be due to irritable weakness of the brain, but neurasthenia a milder "weakness" than with hysteria. The notion that neurasthenia could result from overwork and life stresses made it more palatable, and in some social circles it was even a badge of honor. William Osler, the renowned professor of medicine at Johns Hopkins Hospital in Baltimore, considered neurasthenia as the male hysteria manifested by a state of hyper-reactivity where the man overreacts to the slightest annoyance and finds it impossible to relax [2]. Middle-class businessmen became lucrative clients for many private practices, but the condition was seen in men from all socioeconomic classes. In reality, just as with hysteria, the diagnosis of neurasthenia comprised a variety of nervous disorders, including depression, anxiety disorder, panic disorder, obsessive-compulsive disorder, fibromyalgia, chronic fatigue syndrome, and somatoform disorder.

© The Editor(s) (if applicable) and The Author(s), under exclusive license to Springer Nature Switzerland AG 2021
R. W. Baloh, *Medically Unexplained Symptoms*,
https://doi.org/10.1007/978-3-030-59181-6_4

Freud, the Early Years

When Sigmund Freud entered medical school at the University of Vienna in 1873, he had every intention of entering academic medicine, possibly in the rapidly advancing field of neuroscience. At that time, Vienna was at the forefront of scientific medicine and had many famous scientific researchers. While in his medical training, Freud joined the laboratory of the pioneering physiologist Ernst Brücke with the goal of establishing his scientific credentials. Brücke was known for integrating German laboratory medicine with Viennese bedside medicine. He was one of the founders of the naturalism movement, based on the premise that all living organisms are governed by straight-forward physical and chemical principals, just like inanimate objects. It followed that if one knew the physics and chemistry of the brain, one could understand all behavior, normal and abnormal. While working in Brücke's laboratory, Freud met Josef Breuer, who had already established himself as a promising academic researcher with his work on the neural basis for the self-regulation of breathing (the Hering-Breuer reflex) and on the physiology of the vestibular (balance) part of the inner ear [3]. Freud had expressed a keen interest in the anatomy of the brain, and Breuer encouraged Freud to conduct a series of anatomical staining studies on the root fibers of the auditory (hearing) nerve [4]. But by the time Freud graduated from medical school in 1881, he was in debt, wanted to get married and had all but given up on an academic career. He decided to take a more secure financial position as a doctor at Vienna General Hospital, although he continued to maintain contact with his mentors Brücke and Breuer. Freud became engaged, and after Freud spent a few years in general medicine, Brücke obtained a small grant for him to go to Paris and work with the great Charcot, a last-ditch effort to see whether he might still make an academic career [5]. If not, Freud planned to marry and start a private practice. The timing of his leaving Vienna was auspicious, since there was a growing controversy in the medical community over his experimentation with cocaine, both on himself and on his patients. Freud claimed that cocaine was effective treatment for a wide range of medical conditions, including neurasthenia, and he eventually became an addict. One clear benefit of Freud's experimentation with cocaine was his observation that cocaine was a good local anesthetic. Eye doctors began using it to anesthetize the eye during procedures on the eye.

Freud became enthralled with Charcot after attending a single lecture. He noted that Charcot had an abundance of common sense and ingenuity. The problem was access. Charcot was at the peak of his career, and aspiring neurologists from all around the world flocked to Paris to work under the great man. To gain Charcot's attention, Freud offered to translate Charcot's lecture series into German. This worked beautifully, and Freud soon found himself as part of Charcot's inner circle, with regular invitations to the weekly soirées at Charcot's mansion on the Boulevard Saint-Germain. Freud's time in Paris went by rapidly, and on his return to Vienna he was ready to impress his colleagues with his newfound discoveries. He was particularly enthralled by Charcot's use of hypnosis and the hypothesis that only those with the inherited tendency to hysteria could be hypnotized. However, his Viennese colleagues were not impressed; many of them considered hypnosis to be simply the product of suggestion and subject to fraud and self-delusion. Freud was demoralized and decided to start a private practice and go ahead with his marriage. His associate from Brücke's laboratory, Josef Breuer, had already established himself in a general private practice in Vienna (also for financial reasons) and had many affluent patients, particularly in the Jewish community. He helped Freud establish his new practice, referring patients and providing monetary support. The relationship between Freud and Breuer would be pivotal in Freud's development of psychoanalysis, "the talking cure."

Breuer's Famous Patient, Bertha Pappenheim

Breuer's foray into the field of psychiatry can be directly traced to one of his patients, a bright, young girl who became ill while she was nursing her sick father, whom she adored [6]. She exhibited a range of bizarre neurological symptoms that began with an intense cough followed by attacks of convergence spasm (involuntary turning inward of both eyes), causing double vision. Breuer made a diagnosis of hysteria, and his patient soon developed other symptoms, including facial twitching, and transient right arm numbness and paralysis. Breuer made the chance observation that when his young patient was in a relaxed "autohypnotic state" she would relate the events that occurred at the time a particular symptom began; remarkably, after describing these events, the symptom disappeared. Thus, Breuer arrived at a new treatment method, later called the cathartic method. The philosophical concept of catharsis, a purgation of emotions through art, can be traced back hundreds of years to Aristotle's principal of tragedy. Freud later wrote, "nothing in his education could lead one to expect that he (Breuer) would gain the first decisive insight into the age-old riddle of the hysterical neurosis and would make a contribution of imperishable value to our knowledge of the human mind" [7].

The young girl with hysteria would become the focus of Breuer and Freud's famous book *Studies on Hysteria*, the starting point for the development of psychoanalysis [8]. She was given the pseudonym Anna O. in the book, but Freud's biographer, Ernest Jones, revealed her real name, Bertha Pappenheim, in 1953, much to the consternation of her family and friends. Probably more has been written about Bertha than any other single patient in medical history. It is not entirely clear how Breuer became Bertha Pappenheim's doctor, although most likely he was already the family doctor for the Pappenheims, a prominent Jewish Viennese family.

Bertha seemed to improve with the new treatment method, but after Breuer returned from his summer holidays he found her to be in a "wretched" state, so he again began an intensive daily therapy. He found that when she reported a specific circumstance when one of her many symptoms first occurred, her discussion and description of the circumstance was followed by disappearance of the symptom. With this approach, Breuer systematically achieved an abolition of most of her symptoms. However, the symptoms always came back, and Breuer began to develop doubts regarding the success of his new treatment. He then began for the first time to use hypnosis in an attempt to get Bertha to relive the psychic events leading up to her symptoms. He again noted a dramatic response, although, as before, her symptoms continued to come and go with crisis after crisis.

After working with Bertha over several months, Breuer began to have doubts whether he was the appropriate person to continue her treatment. However, when he attempted to arrange for others to take over her care, she invariably went into a crisis. Finally, in the summer of 1882 Breuer convinced her and her mother that she should be admitted to the Bellevue Sanatorium at Kreuzlingen on Lake Constance. Although no longer involved in Bertha's treatment, Breuer continued to maintain an interest in her case through contacts with the family. Contrary to the impression in *Studies in Hysteria* that Bertha was cured of her illness with Breuer's treatment, she continued to have relapses and was hospitalized on several occasions at the Vienna City Psychiatric Hospital between 1883 and 1887. Even later in life, she continued to have relapsing symptoms, despite becoming a successful writer and working as a social worker.

Breuer didn't tell Freud about Bertha Pappenheim until several months after he stopped treating her [9]. Furthermore, it would be more than a decade before they published her case history in a preliminary communication in 1893 and in the book in 1895. Over the years leading up to the publication of *Studies of Hysteria*, Breuer worked with Freud on numerous patients, but he left the psychiatric aspects to Freud and concentrated on the medical aspects. Why did it take so long for Freud to convince Breuer to go ahead with the publication? Breuer had moved on. He had many other projects, including his vestibular work (which he continued at home mostly in the evenings) and his busy practice. He occasionally saw psychogenic patients, but he referred them to Freud for their care. There is no evidence that he ever used the cathartic treatment method again. Breuer did have concerns that it would be difficult to camouflage Bertha's identity in any publication, but most problematic to Breuer with regard to a joint publication was Freud's developing emphasis on sexuality in his theory on the cause of hysteria. Breuer was aware of and did not disagree with the widely held view that hysteria could result from frustrated sexual desires, but he was uncomfortable with making sexuality the center of their theory on cause. From Freud's point of view, he felt that Breuer's reluctance to publish was connected with the disturbing experience of a sexual attraction that developed between Bertha and Breuer during her treatment. Freud biographer Ernest Jones went even further and suggested that Breuer had developed a countertransference for his patient and that Breuer's wife, Mathilde, suffered from it [10]. He speculated that when Breuer became aware of his feelings for Bertha, he reacted with guilt and broke off the treatment. Bertha reacted to the abandonment by developing a hysterical pregnancy that further horrified Breuer. Jones suggested that Breuer took his wife to Venice for a second honeymoon in an attempt to smooth over the problem. Breuer's biographer, Hirschmüller, could find no documentation of either the hysterical pregnancy or the trip to Venice, but he did feel that Bertha's treatment could have had an effect on Breuer's relationship with his wife.

Freud and Breuer's Book on Hysteria

Studies on Hysteria, published in 1895, had four sections, an overview of the mechanism of hysteria written by both authors, five case histories (Bertha Pappenheim's and four of Freud's patients), a theoretical discussion by Breuer and a discussion of psychotherapy by Freud. The format was highly unusual considering that only the introduction was jointly written. Why even bother to publish jointly? Likely, Freud felt that publishing with Breuer was advantageous, because Breuer discovered the method of treatment and his scientific reputation increased the likelihood of a good reception for the book. To get Breuer's cooperation, Freud agreed to keep the theme of sexuality in the background. Breuer, on the other hand, was loyal to Freud and wanted to support his work, even though he had reservations. The central theme of Breuer's theoretical discussion in the book was "intracerebral tonic excitation" and the need for an organism to maintain constant brain excitation [11]. In a nutshell, he proposed that a "surplus of excitation" gained access to the sensory, vascular and visceral apparatus, causing the observed pathological phenomena. He used the term "conversion" to describe how excitation associated with an emotional idea was converted into somatic symptoms. Over time, the emotion and the idea are dissociated and the "hysterical conversion" is complete. Breuer attributed this concept to Freud, but Freud later wrote that he came up with the name but the concept of conversion was a joint endeavor. In his discussion, Freud focused on psychology, concluding that there were several types of neuroses, including anxiety neurosis, obsessional neurosis and hysteria and that sexual factors were important in the etiology of all of them [12]. Only neurasthenia, which he considered a more restricted neurosis primarily manifested by lack of energy, was not caused by sexual tension. Although each of these neuroses had unique features, he felt that there was marked overlap between symptom complexes. The most severe form of neurosis, hysteria, was usually a mixed neurosis that required different treatments for different symptoms.

In his discussion of psychotherapy Freud indicated that he found it useful to combine cathartic psychotherapy with Mitchell's rest-cure to improve the overall results of both treatments. This is surprising considering the goal of Mitchell's treatment was to avoid thinking and concentrate on relaxing the mind. Freud argued that patients were often bored and daydreamed during the rest cure and rather than interfering with the rest cure the addition of psychotherapy improved the outcome. "A combination such as this between the Breuer and Weir Mitchell procedures produces all of the physical improvement that we expect from the latter, as well as having a far-reaching psychical influence such as never results from the rest-cure without psychotherapy" [8]. As suggested in Chap. 3, Mitchell was very suspicious of psychotherapy and worried that excessive introspection associated with psychotherapy might make symptoms worse than better. Roy Porter made the same point, but more bluntly, when he suggested "Charcot's Tuesday Clinic and the Freudian couch arguably hysterized hysteria, as one might douse a fire with gasoline" [13].

Freud admitted that his "short stories" describing his patients and their response to treatment lacked scientific rigor, but that the nature of the subject was responsible for this, and not his preference. The book received mixed reviews at the time and

Breuer's theoretical discussion was criticized for the lack of specifics, in particular, the lack of a mechanism to explain the excessive brain excitation. Later, Freud speculated that the poor reception of Breuer's section of the book was the main reason Breuer ended their collaboration on hysteria.

Breuer and Freud continued to collaborate on clinical cases, and Breuer maintained an active interest in Freud's developing theories on psychoanalysis, but Breuer did not write any further on psychoanalysis. By the time the book was finally published, Freud had largely abandoned the cathartic method for treating hysteria. The book suggested that the women were cured by the cathartic method but in reality all of them continued to have exacerbating symptoms. Breuer became increasingly uncomfortable with Freud's emphasis on the role of sexuality in the genesis of neurosis and his conclusion that hysteria resulted from a sexual trauma in early childhood. Freud was obviously aware of Breuer's unease, but he continued to seek Breuer's opinion and he needed Breuer's acclamation. Breuer, was an empiricist by nature, a scientist who abhorred broad, sweeping generalizations. He saw nothing as black and white but rather many different shades in between. By contrast, Freud was a dreamer and a zealot. With him it was all or nothing. Criticism of any of his work was taken as criticism of his work as a whole. The final break up occurred in the spring of 1896. In a story handed down by family members, Breuer came across Freud on the street in later years and went to greet him with open arms, but Freud turned away and crossed to the other side of the street [3].

Suppressed Memories and Childhood Sexuality

At the center of Freud's thinking on hysteria and psychogenic illness was the concept of suppressed memories and emotions that somehow lead to physical symptoms. If he could get the patient to recall the repressed memory and the associated emotion, the symptoms might be alleviated. He initially tried Breuer's cathartic treatment and hypnosis, but found these techniques time-consuming and not very effective. He then tried what he called free association, allowing the patient to speak freely, saying whatever came to mind, in the hope that the patient would inadvertently reveal the secrets in the unconscious mind (a "Freudian slip"). But he found that the repressed memories were often kept secret from the conscious mind, and it was up to the therapist to help the patient become aware of the internal psychological conflicts. By carefully listening to the patient, including detailed reports of the patient's dreams, the therapist could help the patient unlock the repressed memories.

A year after publishing *Studies in Hysteria,* Freud published three papers describing his new theory on the cause of hysteria, repressed memories of sexual trauma as a child [14]. Sexual molestations and incestuous assaults were the root cause of hysteria. When prominent members of the Viennese medical community suggested that this was a bit farfetched, Freud expanded his theory to include real or fantasized childhood seductions. This change in his theory was also driven by the disturbing but obvious implication that the fathers of his many affluent women with hysteria were all pedophiles. Even he found that to be unlikely. Freud diagnosed himself and several of his siblings as having a type of hysteria after the death of his father in 1906. Freud became preoccupied with death and experienced numerous gastrointestinal and cardiac symptoms and was convinced that he had a life-threatening cardiac disorder. Was his father a child abuser? Freud was not willing to accept that premise, and he began to gravitate toward a more general theory of the role of sex in psychogenic illnesses.

In 1905 Freud published *Three Essays on the Theory of Sexuality* outlining his new general theory on the central role of sexual drives on psychogenic illness [15]. He introduced the term libido, which represented the energy associated with subconscious sexual urges, a major driving force behind all psychoneurosis. Freud saw childhood development as a series of hurdles, all fraught with potential pitfalls that could create psychopathology. The oral (sucking) and the anal (bowel movements) stages were followed by the phallic stage, the most important stage for the development of repressed desires and fantasies. At this stage, the child becomes aware of its sexual organs as a source of pleasure and develops a profound sexual attraction for the parent of the opposite sex and a hatred for the parent of the same sex (the Oedipus complex). This causes the child to feel guilty and, in the case of a male child, fear retaliation from the father for his sexual attraction toward his mother (leading to castration anxiety). The child must move through a series of conflicts whose successful resolution is required for normal mental health. Psychogenic illnesses resulted from unresolved conflicts.

Freud's Model of the Mind

Almost two decades later, Freud proposed his model of the mind that remains a foundation of modern-day psychoanalysis. He identified three elements of the mind, the id, ego and super-ego. The id consists of instinctual drives like libido; the super-ego is the conscience, largely shaped by one's parents; and the ego is the "self" whose job is to reconcile conflicts between the id and super-ego. The ego resides in the conscious mind, while the id and super-ego are in the unconscious mind, with the superego being a screening mechanism to contain the pleasure-seeking drives of the id. Freud went on to postulate that the ego uses a variety of defense mechanisms to reconcile conflicts, including repression – keeping conflicts in the unconscious; sublimation – directing sexual drives into socially acceptable pursuits such as academic achievement; fixation – staying at one of the developmental stages; and regression – regressing to the behavior of one of the earlier stages of development.

What is one to make of Freud's psychological "theories" in the twenty-first century? There can be little doubt that many of Freud's constructs permeate our twenty-first century vocabulary. Conversion, Freudian slip, free association, libido, ego, repression and sublimation are only a few of the many constructs that the average person recognizes. But do his theories represent a "new science" of the mind and mental illness, as Freud claimed? The answer to that is a resounding no. A scientific theory must be testable, able to be proven true or false. Freud's theories were mostly belief-based and not testable in true scientific fashion. Similar belief-based theories of the mind were espoused by Plato two millennia earlier. Even more disturbing, Freud considered himself a neuroscientist with basic understanding of brain function and anatomy yet he was proposing a theory of the mind that ignored the brain. If there is one thing that neuroscientists can agree upon, it is that the brain is the mind and the mind is the brain. Freud was certainly aware that psychology was at its root the reflection of underlying brain activity, what Hughlings Jackson called psychophysical parallelism. Further, he admitted that someday the molecular mechanisms of mental phenomena may be identified but his theories would have to do in the meantime. One cannot fault Freud for the limited information about brain function in his time, but one can fault him for convincing several generations of psychiatrists to focus on the mind rather than the brain.

Overall Impact of Psychoanalysis

What was the impact of Freud's new psychoanalysis on treating patients with psychosomatic symptoms? Based on accessibility alone, it was a failure, since only a tiny fraction of the population can afford to pay for the regular lengthy treatment sessions. On top of that, it isn't very effective. Most patients know their symptoms are real, due to some disease. They don't like the idea of being referred to a psychiatrist for "talking therapy," the implication being that their symptoms are just in their head. Psychoanalysis, as portrayed in the popular media, is a man with a beard, smoking a pipe, and sitting thoughtfully while the patient, comfortably lying on a couch, talks about their sex life and dreams. How could this help pain, fatigue or dizziness? Psychoanalysis did have a major impact on the training of psychiatrists in the early twentieth century. In America, Freud's concepts dominated most psychiatry training programs often at the expense of general medical training. The result was that psychiatrists were uncomfortable in treating patients with symptoms such as pain, dizziness and fatigue, the common psychosomatic symptoms. Could they be missing an organic disease? Patients could sense the psychiatrist's unease in dealing with psychosomatic symptoms, and since most patients were already certain that they had an organic disease, the psychiatric treatment was doomed to fail.

Physicians, Patients and Psychosomatic Symptoms

If there is one thing that history teaches us about psychosomatic symptoms, it is that there is a symbiotic relationship between physician and patient. Physicians can influence the symptom complex that patients exhibit, and patients are well aware of the symptoms that their doctor expects. This is not to suggest that doctors and their patients are willfully planning illnesses but rather that the symptom complex can be a byproduct of their relationship. For example, Charcot regularly observed the stereotyped pattern of a hysterical fit in his patients, yet this pattern was rarely seen after his death. Classical hysteria in general became relatively rare by the turn of the 20th century, but it persisted longer in France due to Charcot's influence than in England, where physicians were less tolerant of the bizarre antics. Freud noted an evolution of symptoms in his patients with hysteria as his thinking on neurosis evolved, and late in his life he rarely saw a patient with classical hysteria. In America, Beard's diagnosis of neurasthenia caught hold, and it largely replaced the diagnosis of hysteria. Here we can clearly see for the first time the influence of the lay press on influencing the patterns of psychosomatic symptoms. The concept of Americanitis became intertwined with the diagnosis of neurasthenia, and physician self-help books such as Beard's and Mitchell's and articles in the lay press outlined a socially acceptable symptom complex. Another factor that led to the demise of classical hysteria was improved understanding of brain anatomy and physiology by physicians. Neurologists became adept at distinguishing between symptoms caused by structural brain damage and symptoms caused by psychogenic illness. They could easily recognize numbness and paralysis that did not fit the known anatomical pathways. Patients rapidly recognized this problem and gravitated toward more acceptable subjective symptoms such as pain, dizziness and fatigue. There is a clear trend from motor to sensory symptoms in patients with psychosomatic illness beginning in the twentieth century and continuing up to the present time.

Common Sense Psychotherapy

The idea that suggestibility and hysteria were tightly interrelated phenomena dates back to Charcot's notion that susceptibility to suggestion and hypnosis were unique inherited features of hysteria. In other words, if you could be hypnotized you had hysteria. At about the same time in another part of France, a hypnotherapist at the University of Nancy, Hippolyte Bernheim, came to an opposite conclusion: hypnotism was simply a physiological state of mind with heightened susceptibility to suggestion and everyone was susceptible to hypnosis [16]. Suggestibility was a basic human trait that varied in degree from person to person. The doctor therefore could use suggestion, with or without hypnosis, to treat patients with psychogenic illness. Discussing the patient's problems and making suggestions on how to remedy them was to become the new "common sense" psychotherapy. One of the main proponents of this new psychotherapy was the Swiss neurologist Paul Dubois. In his popular book *The Psychic Treatment of Nervous Disorders,* published in 1904, Dubois outlined his therapy, which used the power of suggestion to convince patients that they would get better. Dubois wrote, "It is necessary from the very start that he (the doctor) should establish between them a strong bond of confidence and sympathy… We practitioners ought to show our patients such a lively and all-enveloping sympathy that it would be really very ungracious of them not to get well" [17]. He emphasized the importance of listening to the patient and never interrupting or appearing to be in a hurry. The physician and patient must develop a bond with the common goal of getting the patient better. A key feature of this type of treatment was that patients did not feel as though they were receiving psychotherapy but rather the doctor was treating their condition like any other organic disease.

Of course, this type of common sense psychotherapy was already being practiced by many physicians in the general practice of medicine throughout the world and would continue to be throughout much of the 20th century. The small-town doctor followed his patients over many years and knew all of their idiosyncrasies. Organic and psychogenic symptoms were treated the same with detailed discussion, followed by reassurance. When patients visited their doctor, they expected to get better and they usually did. I have vivid memories of the general practitioner in the small town in Western Pennsylvania where I grew up in the mid-20th century. He knew and cared for everyone in town (about 300 people), and the vast majority of his time was spent talking with patients. Other than an occasional routine X-ray, blood test or urinalysis performed in his office, tests were rarely performed. Similarly, referral to an outside specialist was a rare occurrence. My mother was a typical example of the patients that he spent much of his time with. She was an admitted "nervous worrier," not unlike many other mothers in our town probably in the spectrum of neurasthenia. She constantly worried that either she or one of her four children were coming down with some terrible illness. Her most consistent symptom was chronic fatigue with lack of energy, not unrealistic considering that she was caring for four children and working full time in the family grocery store. She always looked forward to her monthly visit with the doctor and receiving the vitamin B12 shot that he regularly provided. As the time for her monthly visit neared, symptoms began to appear and her fatigue worsened, but after her visit she was bright and cheerful and ready for another month. Of course, she did not have vitamin B12 deficiency; the injection of vitamin B12 was a powerful placebo. Did the doctor intentionally give her a placebo for what he considered psychogenic symptoms or did he actually believe she had B12 deficiency? After graduating from medical school, I had a nice visit with the doctor, who was then retired, and he really believed that my mother and numerous other women in town that he regularly treated with B12 injections were "low on B12" (even though no blood tests were ever performed). This conviction no doubt enhanced the effectiveness of his B12 treatment. But the family doctor is becoming a relic of the past. In 1989, only about 20% of patients in the United States reported that they were willing to trust the family doctor for their health care. More than 50% of patients indicated that they preferred to select their own hospital rather than the recommendation of their family doctor.

At the turn of the 20th century in America, much of the newly developing subspecialty of psychiatry was enamored of Freud's psychodynamic theories. One of the founding fathers of American psychiatry, Adolph Meyer, although aware and interested in Freud's ideas, championed the cause for "common-sense psychiatry" and "preventative psychiatry" [18]. Meyer received his medical degree at the University of Zurich in 1892, and during his training he spent time abroad with John Hughlings Jackson in London and Charcot in Paris. He emigrated to the United States when he could not get a position in Zurich and after a series of positions in neurology, neuropathology and psychiatry in Illinois, Massachusetts and New York, he became the first psychiatrist-in-chief at Johns Hopkins Hospital in Baltimore in 1910. Meyer taught that it was critical to obtain a comprehensive life history of a patient in order to understand the somatic and psychological aspects of their illness, the psychobiology of illness. He introduced the new concept of mental health prophylaxis with emphasis on early intervention in the family, the workplace and in the community, ultimately leading to the mental hygiene and occupational health movements in the United States. In the famous Phipps Psychiatric Clinic he established at Johns Hopkins, Meyer used clinical and laboratory measurements to study the pre-symptomatic and remission phases of mental illness in addition to the acute phases. He felt that somatic and psychological aspects of an illness should be addressed in an identical manner. Never a strong proponent of psychoanalysis, in his presidential address to the 34th annual meeting of the American Psychiatric Society, Meyer stated, "Those who imagine that all psychiatry and psychopathology and therapy have to resolve themselves into a smattering of claims and hypotheses of psychoanalysis and that they stand or fall with one's feelings about psychoanalysis, are equally misguided" [19].

Alternate Medical Treatments and Suggestibility

Since suggestibility plays such an important role both in the development and treatment of psychogenic symptoms, the therapist's belief in a treatment is important for success. Belief is at the foundation of most alternative medical treatments, so to the dismay of the traditional medical community these treatments have traditionally been effective for psychosomatic symptoms. For example, over the centuries, a variety of practitioners have carried out joint and spine manipulations to treat a wide range of symptoms [20]. Popping a dislocated shoulder or hip joint back into place no doubt had a dramatic impact on the suffering patient and the viewing public. The notion of treating "a-little-bone-out-of-place" became the foundation of an entire medical practice. Lay bone setters were prevalent in England and early America. Well known in England was Sally Mapp, the daughter of a bone setter whose techniques had been developed in her family over centuries. "Crazy Sal," as she was known, toured London from her home in Epson "setting bones and curing diseases." The Gentleman's Magazine wrote in 1736 that Crazy Sal "performed cures in bone-setting to admiration, and occasional so great a resort that the town offered her 100 guineas to continue there a year" [20].

Chiropractic has enjoyed great popularity in the United States. Daniel David Palmer, a grocer in Davenport, Iowa who initially experimented with Mesmer's magnetic healing, performed the first chiropractic adjustment on a deaf janitor in 1895. According to Palmer, the janitor developed the deafness after he felt a pop in his back while working in a cramped area. On examination, Palmer noted a lump in the janitor's spine that he interpreted as a spinal misalignment. He adjusted the misalignment and the janitor's hearing came back. Whether this was the actual series of events is in dispute, since the janitor's daughter later said that her father was telling a joke and when he reached the punch line, Palmer slapped him on the back with a heavy book he had been reading [21]. After that blow, her father thought his hearing improved. Palmer developed the notion that all illness was caused by misaligned vertebrae ("subluxations") that interfered with the transmission of what he called "Universal Intelligence," a kind of spiritual energy that connected the brain to the rest of the body through the spine. Just about any symptom could result from the blocked transmission. He likened the subluxation to a "pinched hose." Palmer later compared himself to Christ, Mohammed, and Smith, all founders of new religions [20]. Despite the fact that there is no scientific evidence that "subluxations" of the spine can cause any symptoms or that manual manipulation can correct "sublux-ations" if they exist, chiropractic manipulations continue to be popular with a large segment of the population, particularly for pain and fatigue. Many chiropractors recommend periodic manipulations to maintain normal health and prevent symp-toms. Interestingly, when patients are surveyed, many prefer the care they receive from chiropractors over that received from medical doctors. Chiropractors usually spend more time with patients than physicians do. They provide simple explana-tions that appeal to many patients, and they take advantage of the remarkable heal-ing power of "the laying on of hands."

Of course, the problem with relinquishing the care of patients with symptoms that may be psychosomatic to alternative medical practitioners is that some of these patients have potentially life-threatening illnesses. Someone with scientific medical training must assess the history and examination. Furthermore, patients are becom-ing more sophisticated in their medical knowledge, and many are unwilling to accept non-scientific belief-based explanations for their symptoms. Physicians must use the powerful tools of suggestibility and reassurance judiciously in the appropri-ate situations. In order to do this, they must take the time to listen to the patient and get to know the medical history. Modern-day clinics where the physician sits at a computer typing and reviewing records while questioning the patient during an allotted 15-min appointment just won't work for these patients. Ordering tests and procedures in place of talking with the patient is like throwing fuel on the fire. A suggestion of a rare disease that might be missed or an incidental finding on a MRI of the brain can be the tipping point that causes a downward spiral in the illness. Is it even possible for modern-day scientifically trained physicians to effectively treat patients with psychosomatic symptoms? Patients certainly pick up on the slightest hint of skepticism shown by the physician. Suggesting that the problem is all in their head is prescription for failure in these patients. Unless the symptoms are taken seri-ously, there is no chance for successful treatment. Psychosomatic symptoms are just like any other brain symptoms.

War and Psychogenic Illness

Although even in the early 20th century some physicians still considered hysteria a female disorder, the largest documented epidemic of hysteria in the history of the world occurred almost exclusively men. In World War I, the initial use of the term "shell shock" was for a physical brain injury that merited an honorable discharge and potential war pension [22]. But early in the war it became apparent that many soldiers were experiencing a range of symptoms similar to those reported by patients with shell shock but had not been anywhere near a shell explosion. Symptoms included generalized trembling and shaking, paralysis, visual loss, ringing in the ears, dizziness, headache, confusion, difficulty concentrating, loss of memory and impaired sleep. There were many opinions within the medical community to explain these symptoms. Some suggested subtle microscopic brain injuries such as tiny tears or hemorrhages triggered by nearby blast waves, but how to explain the many cases that were nowhere near an explosion. Over time most felt that traumatic stress and suggestibility were at the root of the symptoms. The mind was enfeebled by fear and emotional stress so that it was susceptible to autosuggestion. Many neurologists and psychiatrists in America, England, France and Germany came to the conclusion that most cases of shell shock were simply male hysteria. The chief consultant in psychiatry with the American Expeditionary Forces in France, Thomas Salmo, pointed out that often the soldiers' hysterical symptoms correlated with their war experiences [23]. For example, a soldier developed blindness after witnessing his buddy blasted to pieces or a soldier developed deafness after hearing unbearable cries for help from wounded comrades. Of course, there were still some physicians who thought that the soldiers were simply malingering to get out of harm's way and that they deserved harsh treatment rather than sympathy and a discharge.

Since hysterical symptoms were thought to be the product of suggestion, the soldiers had to be persuaded to abandon them [24]. The notion a weakness of the will and even outright fakery was common among commanding officers, particularly the generals. Surprisingly, shell shock was more common in officers than in enlisted men or at least officers were treated more often than enlisted men. Heavy losses on the battlefield and the need for replacements no doubt influenced the aggressive treatments inflicted on these men with shell shock. Although traditional treatments such as hypnosis and psychotherapy were reported to have some success, the most common therapy used by French and German doctors was a combination of strong suggestion and electrotherapy. The German physician Fritz Kaufman developed the so-called "Kaufman cure," consisting of a combination of electricity and forced military drill accompanied by loudly shouted orders. Soldiers with paralysis received repeated painful electrical impulses to the paralyzed limb until they gave up and began to move the limb. In Vienna, doctors applied electrical shocks to the mouth and testicles of soldiers with shell shock, while other soldiers watched and waited their turn. In France, the neurologist and neurosurgeon Clovis Vincent organized a re-education camp along the banks of the Loire. Soldiers were shocked, threatened and abused until they gave up on their psychogenic symptoms. Vincent, who was known for his force of personality, would do whatever it took to break the soldier's will. He used extra-large electrodes to deliver a massive current to the soldier's body. After the war, doctors on the winning side were largely forgiven for their ruthless behavior, but in Germany some soldiers and their families sought revenge, and several neurologists were chased from their offices.

The variety of psychiatric symptoms reported by soldiers in WWII were similar to those of soldiers in WWI, but as was occurring in the civilian population over time there was a trend toward fewer motor symptoms and more sensory symptoms [25]. Classical hysteria (by then called conversion reaction) with paralysis and fits was unusual, whereas more subtle symptoms such as visual blurring, back pain, dizziness and hearing impairment were more common. It was not uncommon for the symptom profile to fit the soldier's type of field duty. For example, members of the air force would develop blurring of vision, impaired depth perception or diminished night vision, which would disqualify them from flying but otherwise not be disabling. A sharpshooter might develop visual blurring just in his shooting eye. As occurred in WWI, the soldier's complaints sometimes correlated with his battle experience. For example, a 23-year-old infantry staff sergeant developed paralysis and numbness of the right arm below the elbow, stammering speech and loss of vision while fighting in Italy. When he was examined, there was no evidence of organic weakness or visual loss, and he was reassured and told that he would recover. After rest and further assurance, he rapidly regained the right arm strength and the speech impairment and visual loss disappeared. The soldier reported the following:

> I was with the Armed Div. riding tanks – three of my men got killed by shells then just this side of Rome. We took Grossetto – took a hill, man hit me with a rifle butt that scarred me – I killed him with a bayonet – that bothered me, my father taught me never to kill – he's an invalid; he's a Christian man too.... [W]alked some more, kept going north into the mountains. Got pinned down, shelled for 2 hours, killed two of my men and lieutenant. Got to a little town; Battalion Commander lost his head, ordered four men in; he got nicked and ordered us to withdraw. Then went on tanks that shelled us [weeps], killed my lieutenant...platoon leader was hit, I was in charge. I ordered my men out. I stopped to take one more shot. I heard the Germans holler FIRE in English and that's all I remember until they picked me up in a jeep. My gas mask and shoulder straps had been shot off. Then I went to sleep and I don't remember anything until this morning. The gun was blown out of my hand, and all that was left was the trigger part. I guess the flash must have blinded me. [26]

Another unique feature of WWII was the all-out attack on civilian populations. Including the Holocaust, the number of civilian deaths far exceeded the number of military deaths. Furthermore, civilians were exposed to massive shelling and bombing unlike anything that had happened before. Overall, people with psychosomatic symptoms were largely ignored, since the governments were focusing their resources on the military, and it was in their best interest to paint a picture of a healthy population doing their part in the war effort. Hospitals and clinics were understaffed and patients quickly learned that they provided little help. However, delayed effects of war stress affected a large part of the population and resulted in a wide range of symptoms in later years. After WWII these delayed effects of war stress were studied for the first time. The American psychiatrists Grinker and Spiegel provided a detailed description of 65 soldiers with psychogenic illnesses in their book, *Men and Stress,* published near the end of the war in 1945 [27]. In the book, they separated acute symptoms occurring in combat from delayed symptoms developing after combat. The delayed psychogenic illness was called war neurosis and included psychosomatic states, depression, aggressive and hostile reactions and even psychotic-like states [28]. This set the stage for what later would become post-traumatic stress disorder (PTSD).

PTSD, the Prototypical Delayed Stress Disorder

With the Korean and Vietnam wars, the basic principles of treating soldiers with psychosomatic symptoms in the forward area was well established, and the percentage of soldiers with disabling acute psychogenic illnesses was relatively small compared to World Wars I and II. On the other hand, the percentage of soldiers with delayed combat effects, including developing psychosomatic symptoms, alcoholism and drug abuse, was relatively high. It was estimated that a quarter of all Vietnam veterans required some type of psychological intervention [29]. The syndrome initially called the post-Vietnam syndrome and then post-traumatic stress syndrome (PTSD) consisted of three basic features: (1) flashbacks and dreams of the distressing combat event; (2) loss of emotion and avoidance of situations reminiscent of the traumatic event; and (3) a constant state of increased arousal (anxiety). The history of how our understanding of PTSD has evolved over the years provides good insight into the problems with classification of psychogenic illnesses based on symptoms [30].

After WWII it became apparent that psychiatrists from around the world had major differences in training and conceptual framework with regard to psychogenic illnesses. Symptoms such as those of PTSD were well recognized but were given a variety of diagnoses, including shell shock, combat fatigue, battle stress and traumatic war neurosis. There was a clear need for uniformity in diagnostic criteria, and the fledgling American Psychiatric Association published their first Diagnostic and Statistical Manual (DSM-I) in 1952. This manual, which was largely based on expert consensus (committees of psychiatrists), became the "bible" for the practice of psychiatry in the United States and much of the world and remains so up to the present time. The 1952 manual included a diagnosis called "gross stress reaction," defined as a stress disorder resulting from exposure to extreme physical or mental stress. The disorder had to occur in an otherwise normal person, and it had to subside within weeks or some other diagnosis should be considered. The diagnosis of gross stress reaction was of limited use, and indeed it was dropped from the first revision, DSM-II published in 1968. At the same time, the Vietnam War was heating up and more and more soldiers were being identified with chronic stress disorders. Yet these soldiers were returning home to a hostile environment where the war was extremely unpopular and their combat efforts were unappreciated. This and the lack of appropriate treatment facilities were a formula for disaster, and many veterans harmed themselves and family members. As the diagnosis of post-Vietnam War syndrome became more and more apparent in veterans in the 1970s, PTSD was introduced as a diagnostic category in DSM-III, published in 1980. In contrast with the original gross stress reaction diagnosis, there is typically a delay in the onset of PTSD after the stress and the condition tends to follow a chronic course.

Framers of the initial PTSD definition conceived of the stress necessary to cause the disorder as a catastrophic event, outside the realm of normal human experience. This feature of placing great importance on the causative agent was unique to psychiatric diagnoses. But what is catastrophic stress to one person may not be to another person. Clearly, during the Vietnam War most people exposed to traumatic events did not develop PTSD. How was PTSD different from other psychiatric disorders, such as anxiety disorder and depression? Does a diagnosis of PTSD require the person to be normal prior to the being exposed to stress, and how does one define normal? Wouldn't someone with an underlying illness such as anxiety and depression be more susceptible to PTSD? The answers to these questions remain unclear, despite several revisions of the DSM and refinement in the definition of PTSD.

In the most recent revision, DSM-5 in 2013, a catastrophic event is described as actual or threatened death, injury or sexual violence to oneself or to a loved one. Even indirect exposure such as hearing about a horrific accident might be considered a catastrophic event. In DSM-5, PTSD is not just a fear-based anxiety disorder, as implied in DSM-III and DSM-IV, but rather a trauma and stress-related disorder requiring that the onset is preceded by an adverse environmental event. The same triad of symptoms mentioned earlier is still characteristic, but the symptoms must last for at least a month before PTSD can be diagnosed (a complete reversal from DSM-I criteria).

Since its initial description in DSM-III in 1980, PTSD has become associated with a range of life traumas from military combat to natural disasters, terrorist attacks and physical or sexual assaults. It has become one of the most common psychiatric diagnoses causing a major personal and societal burden. As many as 10% of people in the United States suffer from PTSD. Complicating matters, most of these people meet the diagnostic criteria for at least one other psychiatric diagnosis, particularly depression and anxiety disorder. They have increased rates of surgery, more co-morbid medical conditions and undergo more medical procedures than the general population. They go from physician to physician and yet they often end up frustrated with the system. Current treatment consists of a combination of cognitive behavioral therapy and drugs, such as the selective serotonin reuptake inhibitors, which will be discussed in Chap. 10.

Relationship Between PTSD and Mild Traumatic Brain Injury (MTBI)

With more recent wars, there has been a strong interest in the role of traumatic brain injury (TBI) in post-traumatic psychosomatic symptoms. Blast injuries from high-velocity explosions are very common. Soldiers exposed to these modern explosions suffer a range of symptoms from memory loss and amnesia to anxiety and depression. No doubt some of the symptoms are due to structural brain damage, while others are psychogenic, secondary to the fear and stress associated with the combat environment. When there is a loss of consciousness and gross neurological signs, most would agree that structural brain damage occurred, but what about soldiers who develop symptoms after a blast without loss of consciousness or gross neurological signs? Could they have suffered subtle structural changes in the brain that somehow lead to symptoms? In recent years, the concept of mild traumatic brain injury (mTBI), a brain injury that is bad enough to cause symptoms without obvious neurological findings, has become popular. Although called mild, the effect on the injured person and their family can be anything but mild.

Many soldiers returning from Afghanistan and Iraq complained of a range of chronic symptoms including memory impairment, dizziness and imbalance, head-aches, and difficulty with decision-making [31]. Some of these soldiers had suffered concussions associated with roadside explosions, while others were nearby but not close enough to be concussed. Most were nowhere near an explosion, at least when the symptoms began. Complicating matters further many developed chronic symp-toms lasting more than a year. How should the Department of Defense and the Veterans Administration deal with these soldiers? Should they receive long-term disability, and how should they be treated, as brain injured or psychogenic? This is not a small problem, since more than 25,000 soldiers from Afghanistan and Iraq were diagnosed with mTBI and soldiers continue to be screened for the diagnosis at VA hospitals. Furthermore, older veterans dating back to the Vietnam War who were diagnosed with PTSD may meet the criteria for mTBI. The financial implications could be enormous. There has been a clear change in how soldiers with possible TBI are dealt with at the field level. A soldier exposed to a blast is evaluated by field medics with a standardized questionnaire that includes questions about loss of con-sciousness, amnesia and memory loss. Those with symptoms are given rest and observed for neurological symptoms and signs. Furthermore, officers are instructed to watch for soldiers displaying poor marksmanship, slow reactions, impaired con-centration and unusual behavior. Soldiers with multiple TBIs have to be removed from combat because the risk of post TBI symptoms and later onset degenerative brain diseases increases with the number of TBIs.

How does an explosion cause brain injury? Obviously, if the soldier is thrown to the ground or against some nearby structure, the brain could be injured by blunt force trauma. But what about an explosion nearby that does not lead to head trauma? In the past, it was thought that shock waves from an explosion mostly damaged air-filled structures such as the lungs and bowels. The brain is relatively protected by the hard, thick skull and, in the case of soldiers, by a helmet. But with recent studies in animals, it has become apparent that if the force associated with a nearby blast is large enough, there can be small tears in the deep brain structures caused by dis-placement of the brain within the skull. Shock waves may make their way into the brain through the torso and large blood vessels feeding the brain. In addition to structural changes in the brain, TBI results in alterations in neurotransmitter and hormone production and release, just as occurs with chronic stress, blurring the distinction between organic and psychosomatic post-traumatic symptoms [32].

A variety of symptoms occur immediately after a TBI, including loss of con-sciousness, amnesia, disorientation, confusion and loss of smell. As a broad general rule, the severity of immediate symptoms correlates with the severity of head trauma. If the loss of consciousness is less than 30 min, amnesia is less than 24 h and neurological findings are minimal, the TBI is considered mild (mTBI), although this is an arbitrary cut off and does not reliably predict who will go on to develop chronic symptoms. The most common chronic symptoms after a TBI include fatigue, headaches, memory loss, poor attention/concentration, sleep disturbances, dizziness/loss of balance, irritability-emotional disturbances and feelings of depression. This combination of chronic symptoms has traditionally been called post-concussion syndrome, regardless of whether or not the person lost consciousness. Although TBI and post-concussion syndrome are often interrelated, it is important to note that TBI refers to a type of brain injury, while post-concussion syndrome refers to a grouping of symptoms that occur after a TBI. They are not the same thing. In fact, post-concussion syndrome is a misnomer, since the term syndrome refers to a set of symptoms that occur together, evolve in a characteristic pattern and respond to the same treatment. Epidemiological studies of post-concussion symptoms have found little evidence for a coupling of symptoms, maintenance of symptoms or common response to treatment [33]. In fact, the chronic symptoms after TBI are not reliably predicted by the acute symptoms, and a wide variety of methods are required for treatment. Furthermore, somatic and psychosomatic symptoms are not linked and cannot be reliably predicted by the severity of the TBI. The poor predictability between the chronic symptoms and the TBI no doubt reflects the range of mechanisms of brain injury (focal or diffuse, structural or chemical) and individual genetic and psychosocial factors. Recent prospective studies in athletes who are regularly exposed to TBI and concussions have found that post-concussion symptoms persisting beyond 3 months are as well predicted by pre-concussion psychosocial factors as by the nature or severity of the TBI [34].

The elephant always in the room when discussing psychosomatic symptoms is whether the patient could be malingering, faking the symptoms. The possibility of secondary gain becomes particularly relevant when considering post-traumatic symptoms, since there may be disability payments, pensions and lawsuits pending. Furthermore, the symptoms may be a soldier's ticket out of the combat zone. In Germany just before WWI, there was an outbreak of so-called "pension neurosis" after the government passed a law that provided pensions for victims of railway and industrial accidents who developed mental and nervous debilities. With the onset of WWI, the German government was determined to prevent a similar outbreak of war neurosis, so they supported an aggressive, unsympathetic treatment of shoulders with shell shock. Follow-up studies of people with post-concussion symptoms consistently show that those with compensation claims have more and longer-lasting symptoms than those without compensation claims. Most people agree that malingering is relatively rare when dealing with post-traumatic symptoms, and it should be considered only if there are clear functional or examination inconsistencies with the claimed disability. If one believes the premise that all behavior is the product of environmental history and genes (see Chap. 5), it really doesn't matter whether the patient is intentionally or unintentionally experiencing symptoms. The same argument could be made for all psychosomatic symptoms. Whether intentional or unintentional, the behavior is maladaptive, and patients should be encouraged to get better. Rather than providing negative feedback with long, drawn out adjudication processes, compensation claims must be settled rapidly and positive feedback should be provided to return to normal activities and, whenever possible, to work. Educating patients on post-concussion symptoms and establishing individual realistic goals for return to exercise and employment are an important part of the management. Others, including family, friends, employers and insurers, should be brought into the process, because they can reinforce the goals and provide further positive feedback.

Psychosomatic Medicine

From its inception in the early 20th century, psychoanalytic trained psychiatrists dominated the subspecialty of psychosomatic medicine. One of the founding fathers credited with first using the term psychosomatic medicine in 1922, Felix Deutsch trained with Freud in Vienna and became his private doctor when Freud developed cancer of the throat. As with many other Jewish physicians in Vienna, prior to World War II Deutsch migrated to America, where he became the first professor of psychosomatic medicine at Washington University in St Louis. Deutsch felt that emotional factors were not only important for hysterical symptoms but also for symptoms associated with any chronic organic disease [35]. He considered Breuer and Freud's concept of conversion to be at the root of all psychosomatic symptoms. The mid-twentieth century saw the "psychosomatic movement" flourish in America; the first chapter of the main textbook used by medical students, *Osler's Principles and Practice of Medicine*, was devoted entirely to psychosomatic medicine. Deutsch boasted that psychosomatic medicine deserved to be called psychoanalytic medicine. Like Freud, the pioneers in psychosomatic medicine believed that psychodynamics were the "basic science" of psychiatry.

Another founding father of psychosomatic medicine, Hungarian-born Franz Alexander moved to the Chicago Institute of Psychoanalysis in the 1930s with the goal of performing objective "scientific" studies on psychoanalytic treatment of psychosomatic symptoms. Like Deutsch, he had close ties with Freud, having performed psychoanalysis on Freud's son, Oliver. Alexander's book, *Psychosomatic Medicine*, published in 1950 became a standard in the field [36]. At the Chicago Institute, Alexander focused on identifying the psychological profile of patients with seven chronic organic diseases that he thought had a major psychosomatic underpinning: duodenal ulcers, ulcerative colitis, asthma, essential hypertension, rheumatoid arthritis, thyrotoxicosis and neurodermatitis. The basic premise was that chronic emotional stress associated with a specific psychological profile could build up over time, eventually leading to chronic organ damage. He identified seven distinct psychological patterns one for each disease and attempted to devise treatment strategies for each profile. The profile with duodenal ulcers was difficulty gratifying oral dependency needs and accepting help from others because of shame and guilt, so the patient responded best to authoritative management. Alexander suggested that the therapist could decide what was the best way to reconcile the conflict between the personality and environment, by changing the person or their environment. For example, "the hard-driving business executive, ready to take on more and more responsibilities, who is married to an infantile, demanding, clinging-vine type of wife, may more easily relieve his chronic ulcer symptoms by resolving this marital incompatibility by a divorce and by marriage with a maternal type of woman, than by a prolonged analysis which tries to reduce his 'orality.' He may bear his professional responsibilities without somatic symptoms if he is relieved on one front—namely, in his personal life—from the excessive demands of a non giving wife" [37]. By contrast, patients with asthma had a deeply rooted fear of rejection because of a disturbed mother-child interaction, so the therapist should be uncritical, permissive and understanding. Alexander emphasized that although these psychological profiles were reliably seen with each disease, the same profiles could also be seen in people without disease. He speculated that the specific emotional stress situations only caused disease in people who had an organ vulnerability that was acquired early in life or on a genetic basis. In his later years, Alexander moved to Los Angeles, where he conducted research at the Psychosomatic Research Institute at Mount Sinai Hospital. He attempted to study emotional stress under realistic circumstances by using commercial films that illustrated the interpersonal stress situations common to each of the seven different diseases and carefully monitoring physiological function such as blood pressure, respiration, heart rate and sweating while patients watched the films. Alexander argued that "knowing the special emotional vulnerabilities of patients suffering from different diseases enables us to approach their conflicts more directly, without having to discover anew the nuclear conflict in each case" [38]. Alexander's work is best summarized by his concept of the corrective emotional experience. "The patient, in order to be helped, must undergo a corrective emotional experience suitable to repair the traumatic influence of previous experiences. It is of secondary importance whether this corrective experience takes place during treatment in the transference relationship, or parallel with the treatment in the daily life of the patient" [39]. This concept fell into disrepute with psychoanalysts in the latter twentieth century but has been revived with modern cognitive behavioral therapy, internet-based therapy and self-psychology (see Chap. 10).

Although psychiatric-trained physicians dominated the field of psychosomatic medicine from its inception, a medically trained physician who later developed an interest in psychoanalysis, George Engel, argued that the best way to influence doctors caring for patients with psychosomatic symptoms was through a medical identity rather than a psychiatric identity. Engel was trained in internal medicine, and after showing an interest in psychosomatic medicine he was offered a joint appointment as assistant professor in internal medicine and psychiatry at the University of Rochester Medical School. While there he spent time with Franz Alexander in Chicago studying psychoanalysis. Engel became well known early in his career for a seminal study with Franz Reichsman on the effects of emotional stress on gastrointestinal secretions in a young girl, Monica, who was hospitalized at Rochester Strong Memorial Hospital with esophageal atresia (stricture) for more than a year [40]. The child had a chronic fistula in her stomach and when in the presence of strangers would develop depression withdrawal behavior, whereas with her favorite visitors would show great pleasure. Engel and Reichsman showed that secretions in the stomach markedly decreased during the depression phase, while they increased during the pleasure phase. Engel studied patients on the medical wards and observed a high incidence of separation and depression occurring prior to the onset of their medical illness. The majority experienced a significant change in a relationship and reported feelings of helplessness (stress) within the weeks and months prior to the onset of the illness. He speculated that these psychic reactions to unresolved loss altered biological systems that led to the disease [41]. He rejected Alexander's notion of a specific psychological profile for different diseases but rather postulated a non-specific psychological situation which he called "giving up – given up" that triggered helplessness and hopelessness that contributed to the onset of a somatic disease [42]. The psychological situation caused yet-to-be-determined physiological and biochemical changes when the necessary predisposing factors were present. Like Alexander (and Charcot and others), Engel felt that predisposing biological factors including environmental and genetic were required for the psychic events to cause a specific disease. When a person gives up, they become more susceptible to pathogenic factors in the external and internal environment.

Despite the great promise of the new psychiatric subspecialty of psychosomatic medicine in the mid-twentieth century, by the end of the century there was a general consensus that the subspecialty was floundering and that it was having a relatively minor impact on the overall practice of medicine [43]. As psychiatry moved away from a primary focus on psychoanalysis toward a biological, pharmacological focus, psychosomatic medicine with its strong underpinning of psychoanalysis seemed less relevant. Furthermore, with the improved understanding of the disease mechanisms of organic diseases such as duodenal ulcer, asthma and thyrotoxicosis, the idea that an underlying personality disorder could be important in the disease process seemed less likely and even foolish. Imagine the poor patients with asthma being told their disease was caused by their relationship with their mother! Having episodes of smothering, and being unable to catch your breath could change anyone's personality. Not surprisingly, many patients react negatively to even the suggestion that they should see a psychiatrist for their somatic complaints.

In contrast to psychiatry in the latter twentieth century, the biomedical model for the general practice of medicine seemed to be on solid ground. After all, it was based on sound scientific principles, it had made remarkable technological advances and new treatments were being discovered on a routine basis. For example, with the discovery that bacteria cause duodenal ulcers, most patients were cured with a course of antibiotics (see Chap. 7). Was psychiatry being left behind? In a 1975 commentary published in the *Journal of the American Medical Association (JAMA)*, psychiatrist Arnold Ludwig lamented that much of psychiatry had become "a hodgepodge of unscientific opinions" and that "there can be only one sound foundation for psychiatry, that based on the medical model" [44]. In defending the biomedical model, he pointed out that "those who would argue that the unique contribution of modern psychiatry to medicine is its emphasis on the whole individual rather than on organ pathology and disease process ignore the entire idealistic tradition of medicine. Humanism and belief in the basic dignity of man are not the monopoly of psychiatry. They are value systems embraced by all true physicians" [45]. But how well was the biomedical model working for the average patient with common symptoms such as pain, fatigue and dizziness? Not very well. Modern medicine left little time for physicians to get to know their patients, and the test-first mentality often caused them more harm than good.

In a groundbreaking article published in the journal *Science* in 1977, George Engel argued that a new model for medicine was needed, a biopsychosocial model [46]. He emphasized that all of medicine was in crisis and that the biomedical model of disease was not adequate for medicine or psychiatry: "Medicine's crisis stems from the logical inference that since 'disease' is defined in terms of somatic parameters, physicians need not be concerned with psychosocial issues which lie outside medicine's responsibility and authority" [46]. But since psychosocial factors interact with somatic factors in determining the onset, severity and course of all disease, it is impossible to consider one without the other. Focusing just on the biological abnormality may not restore the patient to health. Even if the abnormality is corrected, psychological and social factors can prolong the illness. Engel noted, "The boundaries between health and disease, between well and sick, are far from clear, for they are diffused by cultural, social and psychological considerations. The traditional biomedical view, that biological indices are the ultimate criteria defining disease, leads to the present paradox that some people with positive laboratory findings are told that they are in need of treatment when in fact they are feeling quite well, while others feeling sick are assured that they are well, that they have no 'disease'. A biopsychosocial model which includes the patient as well as the illness would encompass both circumstances" [47]. Engel expressed some optimism that medical schools around the country were beginning to train physicians using the new model and that young physicians were open to learning about the psychosocial dimensions of illness, but he worried that not much will change unless those who control medical resources buy into the need for a change. Unfortunately, more than two decades into the twenty-first century, there has been relatively little indication that such changes in medical care will happen. Perverse incentives that reward tests and procedures including surgery at a markedly higher monetary rate than talking with patients are the rule rather than the exception in "modern biomedicine."

In Brief

There can be little doubt that Sigmund Freud had a major impact on the public's perception of psychosomatic illnesses, yet his model of the conscious and unconscious mind had relatively little impact on the treatment of psychosomatic symptoms. Overall, psychoanalysis is not very helpful for treating psychosomatic symptoms, and it is not available to the vast majority of people. On the other hand, common-sense psychotherapy based on positive suggestion, reassurance and stress management has proven very effective in a wide variety of settings. The major wars of the twentieth century provided a dramatic example of the effects of chronic stress on the health of human beings. Late in the century, the new medical subspecialty, psychosomatic medicine, documented the importance of chronic stress for most medical conditions including hypertension, heart disease and even cancer. The result was a new biopsychosocial model of medicine. With this historical context, we can now address the biological and psychosocial factors that cause psychosomatic symptoms.

References

1. Showalter E. Hystories. Hysterical epidemics and modern media. New York: Columbia University Press; 1997. p. 4.
2. Shorter E. From paralysis to fatigue: a history of psychosomatic illness in the modern era. New York: Free Press; 1992. p. 22.
3. Hirschmüller A. The life and work of Josef Breuer: physiology and psychoanalysis. [Transl of "Physiologie und Psychoanalyse in Leben und Werk Josef Breuers" Verlag Hans Huber, Bern und Stuttgart, 1978.]. New York: New York University Press; 1989. p. 108.
4. Wiest G, Baloh RW. Sigmund Freud and the VIIIth cranial nerve. Otol Neurotol. 2003;23:228–38.
5. The letters of Sigmund Freud, selected and edited by Ernst Freud. New York: Basic Books; 1960.
6. Hirschmüller A. The life and work of Josef Breuer: physiology and psychoanalysis [Transl of "Physiologie und Psychoanalyse in Leben und Werk Josef Breuers" Verlag Hans Huber, Bern und Stuttgart, 1978]. New York: New York University Press; 1989. p. 85–7.
7. Freud S. An autobiographical study. Translated by James Strachey. New York: WW Norton and Company; 1963.
8. Breuer J, Freud S. Studies on hysteria. Vienna, Deuticke, 1895, Translated by James Strachey in collaboration with Anna Freud. New York: Hogarth Press; 1955. p. 276.
9. Baloh RW. Vertigo: five physician scientists and the quest for a cure. New York: Oxford University Press; 2017. p. 63–72.
10. Jones E. The life and work of Sigmund Freud. London: Basic Books; 1961.
11. Breuer J, Freud S. Studies on hysteria. Vienna, Deuticke, 1895, Translated by James Strachey in collaboration with Anna Freud. New York: Hogarth Press; 1955. p. 192–8.
12. Breuer J, Freud S. Studies on Hysteria. Vienna, Deuticke, 1895, Translated by James Strachey in collaboration with Anna Freud. New York: Hogarth Press; 1955. p. 255–60.
13. Porter R. The body and the mind, the doctor and the patient: negotiating hysteria. In: Gilman SL, King H, Porter R, et al., editors. Hysteria beyond Freud. Berkeley: University California Press; 1993. p. 247.
14. Scull A. Hysteria: the disturbing history. New York: Oxford University Press; 2009. p. 146–7.
15. Freud S. Three essays on the theory of sexuality. Translated by James Strachey. New York: Basic Books; 1962.
16. Bernheim H. New studies in hypnotism. Translated by R. S. Sandor. New York: International University Press; 1980.
17. Shorter E. From paralysis to fatigue: a history of psychosomatic illness in the modern era. New York: Free Press; 1992. p. 249.
18. Scull A, Schulkin J. Psychobiology, psychiatry, and psychoanalysis: the intersecting careers of Adolf Meyer, Phyllis Greenacre, and Curt Richter. US Natl Lib Med. 2009;53:5–36.
19. Meyer A. Thirty-five years of psychiatry in the United States and our present outlook. Am J Psychiatry. 1928;85:1.
20. Homola S. Bone setting, chiropractic and cultism. Panama City: Critique Books; 1963. p. 10.
21. Westbrooks B. The troubled legacy of Harvey Lillard: the black experience in chiropractic. Chiropr Hist. 1982;2:47–53.
22. Myers CS. A contribution to the study of shell shock. Lancet. 1915;186:316–20.

23. Salmon T. The care and treatment of mental diseases and war neurosis. New York: National Committee for Mental Hygiene; 1917.
24. Scull A, Schulkin J. Psychobiology, psychiatry, and psychoanalysis: the intersecting careers of Adolf Meyer, Phyllis Greenacre, and Curt Richter. US Natl Lib Med. 2009;53:168–73.
25. Weinstein EA. Conversion disorders. In: Jones FD, et al. War psychiatry, specialty eds. Washington, DC: Office of the Surgeon General at TMM Publications; 1995. p. 383–407.
26. Weinstein EA. Conversion disorders. In: Jones FD, et al. War psychiatry, specialty eds. Washington, DC: Office of the Surgeon General at TMM Publications; 1995. p. 390.
27. Grinker RR, Spiegel JP. Men Under Stress. Philadelphia: Blakiston; 1945.
28. Crocq MA, Crocq L. From shell shock and war neurosis to posttraumatic stress disorder: a history of psychotraumatology. Dialogues Clin Neurosci. 2000;2:47–55.
29. Crocq MA, Crocq L. From shell shock and war neurosis to posttraumatic stress disorder: a history of psychotraumatology. Dialogues Clin Neurosci. 2000;2:53.
30. Friedman MJ. Finalizing PTSD in DSM-5: getting here from there and where to go next. J Trauma Stress. 2013;26:548–56.
31. Bhattacharjee Y. Shell shock revisited: solving the puzzle of blast trauma. Science. 2008;319:406–8.
32. Arciniegas DB, Anderson CA, Topkoff J, McAllister TW. Mild traumatic brain injury: a neuropsychiatric approach to diagnosis, evaluation and treatment. Neuropsychiatr Dis Treat. 2005;1:311–27.
33. Sharp DJ, Jenkins PO. Concussion is confusing us all. Pract Neurol. 2015;15:172–86.
34. Nelson LD, Tarima S, LaRoche AA, Hammeke TA, Barr WB, Guskiewicz K, et al. Preinjury somatization symptoms contribute to clinical recovery after sport-related concussion. Neurology. 2016;86:1856–63.
35. Deutsch F, editor. On the mysterious leap from the mind to the body: a workshop study of the theory of conversion. New York: International Universities Press; 1959.
36. Alexander F. Psychosomatic medicine. New York: Norton; 1950.
37. Alexander F. The development of psychosomatic medicine. Psychosomatic Med. 1962;24:22.
38. Alexander F. The development of psychosomatic medicine. Psychosom Med. 1962;24:21.
39. Alexander F, French TE. Psychoanalytic therapy: principles and application. Lincoln: University of Nebraska Press; 1980. p. 66.
40. Engel GL, Reichsman F, Segal HL. A study of an infant with a gastric fistula. Psychosom Med. 1956;18:374–98.
41. Engel GL. The concept of psychosomatic disorder. J Psychosom Res. 1967;11:3–9.
42. Engel GL. A life setting conducive to illness: the giving-up – given-up complex. Ann Intern Med. 1968;69:293–300.
43. Rose RM. What are we talking about and who listens? A citation analysis of psychosomatic medicine. Psychosom Med. 1983;45:379–94.
44. Ludwig AM. The psychiatrist as physician. JAMA. 1975;234:603–4.
45. Ludwig AM. The psychiatrist as physician. JAMA. 1975;234:604.
46. Engel GL. The need for a new medical model: a challenge for biomedicine. Science. 1977;196:129–36.
47. Engel GL. The need for a new medical model: a challenge for biomedicine. Science. 1977;196:132–3.

Biological Mechanisms of Psychosomatic Symptoms

5

It is not stress that kills us, it is our reaction to it.

Hans Selye [1]

Stress permeates everyone's life, from the stress of driving to work or working in a demanding job to the stress of dealing with a financial or family crisis. Some people constantly feel stress even when environmental stress is minimal. Emotions such as fear, grief, anger, and guilt all can trigger stress. If stress is not managed it can take a toll on the mind and the body and produce a variety of psychosomatic symptoms including pain, fatigue and dizziness. We are just beginning to understand how stress causes these symptoms and how to treat the symptoms. Given that stress exacerbates nearly all known disease processes, managing stress is the foundation for maintaining good health [2].

The Biological Link Between Stress and Illness

There is a complex relationship between stress and illness. Everyone responds differently to stress. A person's genetic background, personality, coping skills and social support system all influence the susceptibility to stress. As suggested in Chap. 1, chronic stress decreases a person's ability to mount an effective immune response. Nearly all measures of immune function diminish with chronic stress [3]. People with immune deficits are particularly susceptible to stress. Many common diseases such as asthma, ulcerative colitis, coronary artery disease, and hypertension are greatly influenced by stress. An asthma attack can be reliably triggered in a susceptible person simply by placing them in situation in which they are unable to cope [4]. Stress can change the amount of insulin required by a patient with diabetes or

R. W. Baloh, *Medically Unexplained Symptoms*, https://doi.org/10.1007/978-3-030-59181-6_5

the amount of L-dopa required by a patient with Parkinson disease. Even cancer is affected by stress [5]. Studies in women show that a diagnosis of breast cancer is more likely if there was a recent loss of a loved one or another traumatic event. In men, lack of satisfying relationships with friends and family increases the risk of prostate cancer. Of course, stress has its most profound effect on psychogenic illness, often being the primary cause [6].

Research scientists define stress as a disturbance in the equilibrium between a living organism and its environment. In the mid-nineteenth century the pioneering French physiologist Claude Bernard introduced the concept that body systems overall function to maintain a constant internal environment that he called the internal milieu. The body maintains the internal environment by a range of compensatory reactions designed to restore a state of equilibrium in response to changes in the environment. For example, the liver breaks down glycogen to produce glucose in the face of decreased blood glucose. An American physiologist at Harvard Medical School, Walter B. Cannon, expanded on Bernard's theory in the early twentieth century, describing the body's effort to maintain a steady state, often called homeostasis. In the process he founded an entirely new field of study, neuroendocrinology. Initially working on digestive disorders, Cannon noted that emotions such as fear and anger interrupted gastric secretions and impaired digestion, whereas happiness and satisfaction improved digestion. To study the phenomena, he applied painful electrical stimuli to anesthetized animals and noted increased secretion of adrenaline into the blood from the adrenal glands associated with increased breathing rate, dilation of the pupils, increased heart rate, and increased circulation to muscles and brain at the expense of the gut. All of these effects could later be reproduced in the same animal by simply injecting adrenaline into the bloodstream. Cannon explained these findings in evolutionary terms, suggesting that these primitive reflexes served the purpose of "survival of the fittest." In 1915, he coined the term "fight or flight," which were the only two options available for primitive prey in the face of a predator [7]. Cannon was so impressed with the similarity of an animal's response to stimulation of the sympathetic nervous system and injecting adrenaline that he erroneously concluded that the neurotransmitter released in the sympathetic nervous system was adrenaline. It was later shown to be noradrenaline, the precursor of adrenaline.

Between the great wars, the first details regarding the anatomy and physiology of the brain emotional centers emerged. The French neurologist Paul Broca, who is best known for his work on localizing language function to the left frontal lobe, first used the term limbic lobe (from the Latin word for border, *limbus*) in 1878 to describe a large arc of the medial (near the middle) cerebral cortex primarily composed of the cingulate and hippocampal cortex. In 1937, the American neuroscientist James Papez published his landmark paper entitled "A Proposed Mechanism of Emotion," in which he described a brain circuit connecting the cerebral cortex and the hypothalamus that later became known as the limbic system, the emotional system of the brain [8]. In his research laboratory at Yale University, Papez injected rabies virus into the hippocampus and followed its path from one group of neurons to another. Rabies virus has the ability to move across neuronal synapses, so by following its path from neuron to neuron one can identify the connections between brain centers. The circuit that Papez initially identified was cingulate cortex to hippocampus to hypothalamus to anterior thalamus and back to cingulate cortex. Papez proposed that unpleasant emotional experiences such as fear produced activity within this emotional circuit. Support for Papez's proposed theory came 2 years later when the American psychiatrist Heinrich Klüver and neurosurgeon Paul Bucy reported that destruction of the hippocampus on both sides in monkeys produced a remarkable syndrome (later to become known as the Klüver Bucy syndrome) characterized by a complete lack of fear [9]. Animals that would normally be afraid of natural enemies such as snakes showed no fear. A few decades later, the syndrome was observed in human patients who suffered damage to the hippocampus on both sides.

The Hypothalamic-Sympathetic-Adrenal Axis

Adrenaline release from the adrenal glands is under control of the sympathetic nervous system reflexively activated by emotional stimuli. The sympathetic nervous system is composed of nerves and nerve ganglia (groupings of nerve cells) outside of the central nervous system that controls the smooth muscle of gut, blood vessels and glands controlling body metabolism (see Chap. 7). The primary neurons for the sympathetic nervous system are located in the hypothalamus, part of the brain's emotion control system, the limbic system. The hypothalamus is also a key brain neuroendocrine center, so that emotions have the potential to affect body organs through activation of the sympathetic nervous system and through the release of hormones.

The hypothalamic-sympathetic-adrenal axis provides an anatomical substrate to explain how stress and psychological emotions can produce somatic symptoms. Fear and stress trigger neurons in the hypothalamus activating the sympathetic nervous system and releasing systemic hormones including adrenaline. This in turn results in a range of symptoms including generalized shaking, agitation, palpitations, sweating, shortness of breath, nausea, abdominal pain, near-faint dizziness, ringing in the ears and difficulty concentrating all symptoms common with psychogenic illness. With chronic fear and stress the symptoms became chronic.

The Hypothalamic-Pituitary-Adrenal Axis

The Hungarian-born Canadian endocrinologist Hans Selye identified another key neuroendocrine component of the stress response. In a paper entitled "Stress and Psychiatry" in 1956, Selye emphasized the importance of the hypothalamic-pituitary-adrenal axis in the body's response to stress [10]. Walter Cannon had focused on the hypothalamic-autonomic-adrenal connection and release of adrenalin with stress, but Selye pointed out that connections from the hypothalamus to the nearby pituitary gland had an equally prominent role in the generation of stress-related neuropsychological symptoms. The pituitary adrenocorticotropic hormone (ACTH) controls the release of glucocorticoids (steroids) by the cortex of the adrenal gland. With stress, the hypothalamus triggers release of ACTH from the pituitary gland which in turn triggers the release of glucocorticoids. Glucocorticoids play a key role in such basic processes as sleep, muscle strength and immune responses, and their release with chronic stress accounts for many of the changes in the brain associated with psychosomatic symptoms.

Stress-related activation of the hypothalamic-pituatary-adrenal axis and release of glucocorticoids explain why many infectious diseases such as tuberculosis are aggravated by exposure to stress and why the rest cure results in faster healing of tuberculous lesions. Animals injected with glucocorticoids are much more susceptible to infections and more susceptible to a variety of medical illnesses including gastric and duodenal ulcers (see Chap. 7). The so-called "stress shift" of pituitary activity is an important consequence of the stress induced increased secretion of ACTH. With the chronic increased secretion of ACTH, the pituitary gland cannot maintain optimal production of other important hormones such as the gonadotrophic hormones (sex hormones). Female rats exposed to physical and emotional stressors stop menstruating, develop ovarian atrophy and during lactation stop milk secretion. Male rats develop involution of the testes. Clinical studies in humans show that stress causes decreased libido and fertility in both sexes accompanied by amenorrhea in women and impotence in men. A classic viscous cycle develops whereby continuous worry and fear causes sexual dysfunction which in turn causes more stress.

Stress and Neuroplasticity

The hypothalamus-autonomic-adrenal and the hypothalamus-pituitary-adrenal connections can explain many of the physical symptoms associated with stress but what about the emotional behavioral symptoms, fear, anger, flashbacks, blunting of emotions and avoidance behavior. Traditional psychiatric concepts such as dissociation, conversion, regression and repression are based on theories of the mind that have no basis in brain anatomy and physiology and provide little insight into what is happening in the brain to explain psychogenic features of stress. Even more important psychoanalytic treatments don't work very well for stress-related symptoms. The limbic system with direct connections to the hypothalamus is a logical substrate for emotional symptoms. Clinical observations in patients show blunting of fear and emotions with damage in the limbic system, but how do these structures control emotions and behavior? How does stress lead to malfunction in these critical brain pathways? For this we need to understand the cellular molecular mechanisms underlying brain plasticity.

A basic feature of all living organisms is the ability to adapt to their surroundings. Even single-cell organisms can respond to noxious stimuli with evasive behavior. Animals with a nervous system modify behavioral responses by modifying the connectivity within their nervous system. In the late nineteenth century, the Russian physician and physiologist Ivan Petrovich Pavlov conducted a series of experiments that revolutionized our understanding of neuronal plasticity [11]. Based on his simple observation that dogs in the laboratory would drool when they saw a lab coat, Pavlov surmised that the dogs associated the lab coat with food because they always received food from someone wearing a lab coat. To prove his theory, he developed a method to measure saliva production and changed the "conditioning stimulus" from a lab coat to a loud noise, ringing a bell. If he rang a bell each time that food was presented after multiple trials the animals would automatically increase salivation when the bell rang even without food. This learning to associate the bell with salivation would dissipate with time after the training stopped but could be reinstated with a brief period of retraining. Pavlov also studied the animals' responses to a noxious stimulus such as a painful shock to the foot. Normally animals rapidly withdrew the extremity, the pupils dilated and the heart rate and breathing rate increased. If a benign stimulus such as a touch or a bell ring was presented immediately after the painful stimulus, the animals had the same response to the benign stimulus as to the noxious stimulus as though the nervous system was hypersensitive to stimuli. If the noxious stimulus was repeated multiple times, the animals gradually decreased their response, a type of habituation. If the noxious stimulus was withdrawn for a period of time and then reintroduced, the animal responded to it as with the initial exposure.

Pavlov surmised that there must be changes in the brain associated with these different types of learning but knowledge regarding neuronal mechanisms was rudimentary at the time. The Spanish anatomist Ramon y Cajal had just formulated the "neuronal theory" based on the idea that nerve fibers (axons) terminated next to the cell bodies of other neurons and not in a latticed network as was generally accepted at the time [12]. Cajal speculated that the junctions (synapses) between the axon terminals and the cell bodies and their branches called dendrites were important for learning within the brain. He suggested that the connections between neurons could be reinforced by multiplication of the axonal terminal branches. Jerzy Kornorski, a Polish neuropsychologist who spent 2 years in Pavlov's laboratory, was the first to use the term plasticity to describe the changes that occurred in the brain with learning. He proposed that neuronal systems were plastic and could change permanently based on the number and combination of incoming signals.

Hebb's Synapse

The field of psychology flourished in the twentieth century but two individuals stood out above all the rest, the Canadian Donald Hebb and the American B F Skinner (discussed later in the Chapter). Hebb's work on the synaptic basis of learning not only changed the course of psychology in his time but it continues to influence neuroscientists well into the twenty-first century. Hebb was born in Nova Scotia in 1904, the son of two physicians [13]. His mother was enamored with the theories of Montessori and schooled him at home until age 8. Hebb was a brilliant student in mathematics and science, but he originally wanted to be a novelist, and his writing skills served him well throughout his career in psychology. As a graduate student in psychology at McGill University, Hebb focused on the nature-nurture controversy regarding intelligence and he speculated that intelligence could be influenced early learning. After McGill, Hebb had further graduate training with the American psychologist Karl Lashley at the University of Chicago and then followed Lashley to Harvard, where they conducted early experiments on learning and memory. Hebb then returned to Canada to work with the famous neurosurgeon Wilder Penfield at the Montreal Neurological Institute for 2 years, followed by a faculty position at Queen's University in Kingston, Ontario. Here he developed IQ tests for rats and humans and provided experimental support for his earlier notion that one's early experience could influence intelligence, a radical idea at the time since most thought that intelligence was innate.

When Lashley became director of the Yerkes Laboratory of Primate Biology in Florida in 1942, he invited Hebb to join him and study the effects of localized brain lesions on emotions and behavior. Hebb was to develop tests to quantify emotions and behavior in chimpanzees. He later told his graduate student Peter Milner that he "learned more about human behaviour during his 5 years observing chimpanzees than he had in any other 5-year period of his life, except the first" [14]. Another benefit of Hebb's stay in Florida was that it allowed him time to read and think about a question that had dogged him since his graduate-school days: How does the brain store thoughts and concepts? The simple notion of a brain where sensory nerves synapse on motor neurons to produce reflex behavior left little room for complex learning and behavior. At that time, he read a paper by the Spanish neurophysiologist Raphael Lorente de Nó describing how sensory signals originating from the semicircular canals of the inner ear were passed on to chains of interneurons in the brainstem that modulated and prolonged the signals on their way to higher centers. Lorente, who trained with Cajal, drew beautiful pictures of the feedback loops of neurons that received the incoming sensory information. Hebb immediately saw these loops of reverberating neurons, which he would later call "cell assemblies," as a potential substrate for storing information such as thoughts and concepts. Analogous to Einstein's "what if" experiments after concluding that nothing could move faster than the speed of light, Hebb systematically questioned how "cell assemblies" could generate ideas, memories, images, thoughts and behaviors. His famous book, *The Organization of Behavior,* published in 1949, outlined his theory of the "cell assembly" and even speculated on how the theory could explain various aspects of psychological illness [15]. A basic feature of the Hebb's cell assembly was what later became known as a "Hebb synapse," when two synaptically connected cells within the assembly repeatedly fired together their synaptic connectivity increased over time. Hebb speculated that growth or metabolic change occurred at the level of the synapse providing the basic building block for learning (plasticity) within the brain. Thoughts and concepts were stored within chains of interneurons whose connectivity was constantly being modified by new sensory experience.

Molecular Mechanisms of Brain Plasticity

Further breakthroughs in understanding brain plasticity would require improvements in technology and molecular biology that only became available in the latter half of the twentieth century. With these techniques, Viennese-born Eric Kandel performed a series of key experiments on neural plasticity in the giant marine snail *Aplysia* that ultimately lead to his receiving the Nobel Prize in Physiology and Medicine in 2000 [16]. Kandel, who fled Austria with his family in 1939 at age 9 and came to the United States, became interested in learning and memory early in his career and planned to be a psychoanalyst. While working as a postdoctoral fellow in the National Institute of Health (NIH) in Bethesda, Maryland, he conducted a series of experiments recording from neurons in the hippocampus of cats. Although he and his colleagues were able to obtain basic information about neuronal firing patterns in the hippocampus, Kandel rapidly became convinced that the system was much too complex to clarify the basic mechanisms of learning. There are billions of neurons in the cat brain and relatively little was known about connectivity between the individual neurons. He concluded that he would need to study a much simpler nervous system to be able to understand how learning occurred. His basic premise, that fortunately proved to be true, was that mechanisms identified in primitive nervous systems would generalize to more complex nervous systems, including the human brain [23].

The brain of the sea snail *Aplysia* consists of about 20,000 neurons located in nine separate groupings or ganglia. With time, Kandel was able to map out all of the neurons and their connections in one of the ganglia, the abdominal ganglia consisting of about 2000 neurons. He focused on one reflex mediated by the abdominal ganglia, the gill-withdraw reflex. Stimulating a point on the skin of the siphon caused the gill to withdraw to protect it from damage. The reflex was mediated by six sensory neurons that relayed the sensation to two interneurons and to six motor neurons that innervated muscles that caused the gill to retract. One cell in the ganglia (R2) was so large (about 1 mm in diameter) that it was easily identified by the naked eye without the need for magnification. He was able to penetrate the neurons with a glass pipet and maintain recordings for many hours. By comparison, the largest neurons in a cat's brain are about 20 micrometers and could only be seen with a high-power microscope and intracellular recordings could only be maintained for a few minutes. By electrically stimulating axons synapsing on R2 from other neurons in the ganglia while recording from R2 he was able to show that all of Pavlov's paradigms (conditioning, sensitization and habituation) could be replicated at the synaptic level. This meant that synapses must physically change with experience.

Kandel studied the cellular basis for learning at the synapse between the sensory and motor neurons in the gill-withdraw reflex. The neurotransmitter released at the sensory-motor synapse was glutamate, which others had already shown to be the main excitatory neurotransmitter in the mammalian brain. Shocking the tail of the animal enhanced glutamate release and synaptic transmission at the synapse for several minutes after the shock – the classical paradigm for sensitization. The tail shock activated interneurons whose axon terminals released the neurotransmitter serotonin (known to be involved in behavioral responses) at synapses on the axon terminals of the sensory neurons. Serotonin receptors in the presynaptic membrane then activated a cascade of intracellular "second messengers" that increased the amount of glutamate released at the sensory-motor synapse. If the animal received a long series of shocks to the tail it produced a much longer sensitization associated with sprouting of new synaptic terminals between the sensory and motor cells. In this case, a second messenger entered the nucleus of the sensory cell activating specific genes to produce proteins for forming new synapses. This process, called long-term potentiation (LTP), is the most studied model of neuronal synaptic plasticity. Early phase LTP does not require new protein synthesis and lasts for up to 3 h, and late phase LTP requires new protein synthesis and lasts for more than 3 h and can last for as long as the animal lives. LTP in the brain is a key factor in learning and memory and provides a mechanism for chronic stress to change the connectivity between different brain centers.

Stress and the Limbic System

The emotional brain, the limbic system, plays a major role in the body's response to stress. Limbic connections from the hippocampus to the hypothalamus activate Cannon's sympathetic-adrenal system and Selye's hypothalamic-pituitary-adrenal axis producing a variety of somatic symptoms described earlier in the chapter. The hippocampus is a critical learning and memory center in the brain and is one of the most plastic regions of the brain. Unlike other organs of the body that are constantly renewing themselves by regenerating new cells from immature stem cells, the brain is relatively stable with very little neuronal turnover. However, in parts of the hippocampus new neurons are constantly being produced from progenitor stem cells, a process that continues throughout life, although diminishing with aging [17]. Both neuroplasticity and neurogenesis are important for learning and behavior and are highly susceptible to stress [18, 19]. Glucocorticoids released from the adrenal cortex during chronic stress activate receptors in the hippocampus producing a positive feedback loop via its connections to the hypothalamus. In animal models, chronic stress impairs neuroplasticity and neurogenesis and shrinks the hippocampus producing an anxiety/depression like state. Drugs such as the selective serotonin re-uptake inhibitor, fluoxetine (Prozac), improve neuroplasticity and neurogenesis and anxiety and depression symptoms [20]. Physical exercise has a very similar effect. These animal studies suggest a central role for neuroplasticity and neurogenesis in psychogenic illnesses and provide a mechanism to explain why certain drugs and exercise relieve the symptoms.

Nerve Growth Factors and Stress

Growth factors are molecules critical for development, differentiation and plasticity of neurons in the brain. Of the four groups of growth factors expressed in the brain, brain-derived neurotrophic factor (BDNF) has been shown to play a critical role in mediating the effects of stress on brain function [21]. BDNF is highly expressed in the hippocampus and the level of expression is very responsive to stress. BDNF appears to be a molecular intermediary for neuroplasticity and neurogenesis in the hippocampus and for therapeutic interventions such as antidepressant drugs and exercise. In rodent models that measure the animal's ability to suppress fear with learning, BDNF plays a key role in fear conditioning, consolidating fear memories and facilitating extinction learning. Slight genetic variants in the BDNF peptide or its receptor, decrease BDNF signaling and increase the risk of developing stress induced psychogenic illnesses including depression, fibromyalgia and post-traumatic stress disorder (PTSD) [22, 23]. BDNF signaling is also influenced by female hormones such as estradiol which could in part explain the increased incidence of stress-related illnesses in women. As we will see in Chap. 10, drugs that target BDNF signaling are potential therapeutic options for psychosomatic symptoms now and in the future.

Proinflammatory Cytokines and Stress

Chronic stress is associated with the increased levels of proinflammatory cytokines released by activated immune cells, macrophages in the blood and microglia in the brain. Cytokines such as interleukins are peptides that control the inflammatory response. They not only alter the immune response but also contribute to the brain effects of stress [24]. In animal models, stress-related release of interleukins impairs neuroplasticity and prevents new synapse formation in the hippocampus. Drugs that block cytokines prevent these antineurogenic effects and the behavioral symptoms of depression caused by stress [25, 26]. Cytokine release with stress in humans induces symptoms of depression including anhedonia and sleep disturbances. Cytokine levels are elevated in the blood of depressed patients and genes that code for cytokines are upregulated in the prefrontal cortex in patients with depression. The combination of glucocorticoid over-reactivity, decreased BDNF signaling, and increased cytokine signaling provides a potent biological triad for depression and other psychogenic illnesses associated with chronic stress.

The Amygdala-Prefrontal Cortex Connection

A key center for stress induced effects on the brain is an almond shaped nucleus deep in the temporal lobe, the amygdala, long known to be important in generating fear and anxiety associated symptoms [27]. As in the hippocampus, BDNF and cytokines are important for mediating fear conditioning in the amygdala. Incoming sensory signals can result in long-term potentiation (LTP) in a subgroup of neurons in the amygdala important for generating fear and anxiety. These excitatory neurons are normally kept in check by inhibitory feedback under the control of the prefrontal cortex, the key center for managing complex cognitive behavior such as planning and problem solving (so-called executive functions). Impaired prefrontal inhibitory control of the amygdala can lead to chronic hypersensitivity and a persistent state of fear and anxiety. The prefrontal amygdala connection is clearly important in cognitive control of emotions and some think it may be the "holy grail" for understanding the mechanism of psychosomatic symptoms. This prefrontal amygdala inhibitory pathway is a good example of Hughlings Jackson's concept of an evolutionary advanced "thinking brain" controlling a more primitive "emotional brain" (see Chap. 3). It is also a potential target for future therapeutic interventions (see Chap. 10).

Central Sensitization, a Model of Neuroplasticity

Since we understand a great deal about how central sensitization to pain occurs, a brief review of the process can provide insight into the mechanisms of psychogenic pain and to psychosomatic illness in general [28]. When pain signals in peripheral nerves arrive at the spinal cord, they trigger the release of the excitatory neurotransmitter, glutamate, which crosses the synapse to activate secondary transmission neurons that carry the pain signals up the spinal cord to the brain. As noted earlier, persistent release of glutamate can lead to the process of long-term potentiation (LTP), a type of neural plasticity whereby more glutamate receptors are expressed in the secondary neurons and new synapses are formed between the primary and secondary neurons. The overall effect is that secondary pain neurons become more sensitive to peripheral pain signals. The process of LTP occurs in the spinal cord and at other pain relay stations in the brain. The result is that any persistent source of pain including minor surgeries can potentially trigger central hypersensitivity to pain. This explains why some surgeons recommend using local anesthetic injections near the site of surgery in addition to general anesthesia during an operation. The barrage of pain signals triggered during surgery can potentially lead to pain hypersensitivity and chronic pain after surgery, even though the patient is unaware of pain while under the general anesthesia.

The Descending Pain Modulatory System (DPMS)

Pain transmission at the level of the spinal cord is normally kept in check by a descending inhibitory pathway originating in the brainstem called the DPMS [29]. The DPMS receives direct input from the spinal cord pain transmission neurons and provides negative feedback by activating spinal cord inhibitory interneurons. The DPMS also projects to the limbic system of the brain and receives feedback from that system modulating the emotional reaction to pain. Endogenous opioids (endorphins) are the main neurotransmitter within the DPMS and the DPMS has the largest number of opioid receptors in the brain. The DPMS provides a mechanism for psychogenic factors to influence pain sensitivity. It is suppressed by stress, depression and anxiety and activated by opioid drugs, relaxation techniques, exercise, acupuncture and placebo treatments. If you believe a pain treatment will work, the DPMS is activated, endorphins are released, and the pain is relieved. The DPMS also plays an important role in stress-induced analgesia. In 1946 the American anesthesiologist Henry Knowles Beecher described how the majority of soldiers that he treated during WW II with major injuries such as compound fractures and penetrating wounds of the chest reported slight or no pain and did not ask for pain medication [30]. He speculated that the strong emotions associated with the injuries somehow suppressed the pain. Similarly, athletes who suffer severe injuries in sport often do not experience pain until the game is over. From an evolutionary perspective reduction in pain during extreme but brief stress makes sense since it allows an animal to react as if there were no pain improving chances of survival. The opposite effect, where chronic stress and anxiety suppress the DPMS and increase pain sensitivity, is maladaptive but commonly occurs with psychosomatic pain disorders.

Stress and Brain Neurotransmitters

As an overview, central sensitization results from increased sensitivity to the excitatory neurotransmitter, glutamate within brain pathways. A variety of other neurotransmitters modulate the degree of central sensitization and provide a mechanism for stress and other psychological factors to influence the sensitization process. For example, as noted in the prior section, release of endogenous opioids within the descending pain modulatory system (DPMS) can inhibit the excitatory transmission at multiple levels within the central pain pathways. The endogenous opioids activate interneurons that release the main inhibitory neurotransmitter, GABA, decreasing excitatory transmission. The monoamines, noradrenaline, serotonin and dopamine modify excitatory and inhibitory transmission throughout the brain and the endocannabinoid system (the system activated by cannabis) modulates the release of all three of these transmitters. Remarkably, slight genetic variations in these transmitter proteins and/or their receptors have been shown to increase susceptibility to stress and development of psychosomatic symptoms. All of these neurotransmitters represent potential drug targets for future treatments of psychosomatic symptoms.

Glutamate

Glutamate is the main excitatory transmitter released in the spinal cord and brain and the glutamate excitatory synapse plays a pivitol role in neuroplasticity and the brain's response to stress [31]. Glutamate is stored in small vesicles in the presynaptic terminals and is released into the synaptic cleft, where it activates three different varieties of receptors expressed in the post-synaptic membrane (AMPA, NMDA, and mGLuR). The relative stimulation and expression of these different receptors controls long-term potentiation (LTP) and learning at the synapse. Another important component of the excitatory synapse, glial cells (astrocytes) containing glutamate re-uptake transporters surround the synapse and control extracellular concentration of glutamate. Overall, several hundred different proteins are involved in the process of excitatory neurotransmission. Animal studies show that all three components of the excitatory synapse (pre-synaptic release, post-synaptic uptake and glial re-uptake) are sensitive to regulation by stress [32–34]. For example, pre-synaptic release of glutamate and the expression and density of post-synaptic receptors and glial re-uptake transporters are altered by glucocorticoids released with chronic stress. Changes in glutamine transmission in the pre-frontal cortex and hippocampus can explain impairments in attention and spatial and contextual memory in rodents after chronic stress. Not surprisingly, the glutamate neurotransmission system is a prime target for new drug development for controlling stress effects on the brain (see Chap. 10) [35].

Gamma Aminobutyric Acid (GABA)

The main inhibitory neurotransmitter in the brain, GABA, plays an important role in modulating the response to stress. GABA is released by interneurons throughout the brain including interneurons in the hypothalamus and GABA can attenuate the response to stress by inhibiting the hypothalamic-pituitary-adrenal axis and the release of stress hormones [36]. On the other hand, chronic exposure to stress decreases sensitivity and availability of GABA receptors which can cause increased response to stress and development of anxiety and depression. Drugs that enhance GABA signaling such as the benzodiazapines (for example lorazepam and diazepam) inhibit the release of stress hormones and improve anxiety and depression. GABA levels are increased after long-term treatment with selective serotonin and noradrenaline reuptake inhibitors and GABA modulates the response of the serotonergic and noradrenergic system's response to stress. Genetic variations in the GABA receptors can increase the stress response and increase the risk for developing psychogenic symptoms [37].

Noradrenaline

The main neurotransmitter in the autonomic nervous system, noradrenaline, is also an important neurotransmitter in the brain for pain perception and anxiety [38]. The locus coeruleus (LC), located in the high brainstem, is the main noradrenergic nucleus in the brain. Neurons in the LC send nerve fibers throughout the brain which play a major role in arousal, attention and pain perception. There are projections to the amygdala and hypothalamus of the limbic system that trigger fear and anxiety associated with threat including activation of the autonomic nervous system. Increased neuronal activity in LC is associated with anxiety and panic attacks, and there is a strong association between chronic pain and chronic anxiety. Furthermore, the LC is a major sleep center, controlling the sleep cycle and different stages of sleep. Impaired sleep enhances stress and anxiety, which leads to further interruption of sleep – a classic viscous cycle.

Serotonin

As noted earlier, Eric Kandel showed that serotonin is an important neurotransmitter in learning in the primitive brain of the giant marine snail, A*plysia*. It also plays a critical role in the stress response. Most serotonin containing neurons are located in the raphe nuclei located at the back of the brainstem near the midline. Neurons in the raphe project throughout the brain, including major projections to key pain centers such as the descending pain modulatory system (DPMS) and to emotional centers in the limbic system. Alterations in brain serotonin levels are associated with chronic pain and the development of mood disorders. Pain and depression are tightly interrelated; pain causes depression and depressed people are more likely to develop chronic pain than people without depression (see Chap. 7) [39]. People with chronic pain have lower pain thresholds, become preoccupied with the pain, and find it difficult to enjoy normally pleasurable activities. Functional MRI studies show that similar limbic brain areas are activated with chronic pain and with depression. The neurotransmitters noradrenalin and serotonin play important roles in both pain and depression. The hallmark of depression is abnormal regulation of these neurotransmitters and drugs that increase brain noradrenalin and serotonin levels are used to treat depression, anxiety and chronic pain (see Chap. 10).

Dopamine

The discovery in the 1950s that degeneration of the brain dopamine system causes the clinical signs of Parkinson disease not only led to an effective treatment with L-dopa (a drug that increases dopamine production in the brain) but also focused scientific interest on dopamine neurotransmission in the brain. It soon became evident that dopamine not only had a role in the control of muscle coordination but also played a key role in behavior such as gambling and addiction and with the painful and pleasurable sensations associated with these behaviors. Some patients being treated with L-dopa developed risk-taking behaviors such as compulsive gambling. Around the same time, researchers at McGill University in Canada reported that when electrodes were placed in the forebrain of rats, the rats would continuously press a bar that triggered electrical stimulation of the forebrain even at the exclusion of all other activities even eating [40]. These areas in the brain became known as the motivation/reward network, and dopamine was shown to be the key neurotransmitter within the network.

The response to sensory stimuli including pain is highly dependent on activity in the motivational/reward network which includes the prefrontal and hippocampal cortices and several subcortical nuclei [41]. There is considerable overlap in the dopamine projections to these cortical and subcortical regions and between the motivation/reward network and the DPMS. Endorphins and serotonin modulate the dopamine signals defining different aspects of the reward such as bliss, thrill and craving. The level of expression of the dopamine receptors in the network determines one's ability to feel pleasure and pain [42]. Dysfunction in the motivation/ reward dopamine network is associated with a variety of clinical syndromes including chronic pain and depression. Investigators at Oxford University in England performed an interesting set of experiments in which they demonstrated how the context in which a painful stimulus is presented markedly influences the experience [43]. They used functional MRI, a technique to measure blood flow to different parts of the brain. Increased blood flow to an area indicates increased nerve firing in that area whereas decreased blood flow means decreased nerve firing. Sixteen healthy individuals were presented a moderately painful stimulus in two different contexts one in which they were expecting an intense painful stimulus and another in which they were expecting a non-painful stimulus. Surprisingly, subjects rated moderate pain as pleasant when they were expecting intense pain despite rating the same pain as painful when they were not expecting a painful stimulus. The "pleasant pain" was correlated with increased nerve firing in motivation/reward centers compared with the "painful pain," where there was decreased firing in these centers. These types of experiments nicely illustrate the importance of expectation on sensory perception and in the next chapter we will address the role of expectation, beliefs and mind set in production of psychosomatic symptoms.

Cannabinoids

The brain endocannabinoid system is another important modulator of the response to stress [44]. The presynaptic receptor, CB1, is heavily expressed in the hippocampus, amygdala and prefrontal cortex and plays a key role in adaptation to stress. Activation of CB1 receptors enhances serotonin and noradrenaline signaling and regulates the sensitivity of the hypothalamus-pituitary-adrenal axis. In animal models, decreasing CB1 expression leads to a heightened stress response and development of anxiety and depression [45]. Normal human subjects given the appetite suppressant, rimonabant, a drug that blocks the CB1 receptor, have a marked increase in anxiety and depression symptoms [46]. Preliminary studies indicate that slight variations in the gene coding for CB1 impair affective sensory processing under stress [37].

Stress and Human Behavior

Like Donald Hebb, the American psychologist, BF Skinner, was also influenced by Pavlov's conditioning experiments. Skinner's work on what he called operand conditioning provided the foundation for behavioral therapy, a major component of current-day treatment of stress-related psychogenic disorders. Skinner was professor of psychology at Harvard from 1948 to 1974 during which time he published key papers and books that influenced thinking about human behavior. In a nutshell, Skinner felt that all human behavior was a result of environmental history and genes; there was no such thing as free will. He argued that scientific methods could be applied to study behavior just as they were used to study other body functions. What one introspectively observed was a byproduct of the physical state of the brain, not some nonphysical entity. He had no time for traditional Freudian psycho-dynamic mind theory. Late in his life he stated,

> For twenty five hundred years people have been preoccupied with feelings and mental life, but only recently has any interest been shown in a more precise analysis of the role of the environment. Ignorance of that role led in the first place to mental fictions, and it has been perpetuated by the explanatory practices to which they gave rise. [47]

Operant Conditioning and Behavioral Therapy

Skinner provided a definition of operant behavior and an outline of how environmental variables controlled behavior in his very first book, *Behavior of Organisms,* published in 1938 [48]. Unlike with classical conditioning behavior described by Pavlov, operant behaviors are "emitted" not induced by a particular stimulus. A person behaves as they do based on the current state of their brain, most of which is out of the reach of introspection. What is introspectively observed, the self, is a "collateral product" of their environmental history. Reinforcement either positive or negative is the main process for shaping and controlling behavior. Skinner argued that both positive (praise) and negative reinforcement (punishment) could ultimately reinforce a behavior. Although punishment is often used to stop a behavior the stoppage is temporary and there can be unwanted consequences. Human behavior is constantly being "shaped" by environmental responses leading to complex behavior, a "chaining" of relatively simple responses. Sometimes superstitious behavior results when an action is followed by positive reinforcement even though it was a chance occurrence unrelated to the behavior. For example, when a gambler blows on the dice before throwing them because he previously won after blowing on the dice. Skinner developed what he called an operant conditioning chamber (others called it a Skinner's box) to study animal behavior in a controlled environment. The box contained a lever that the rat or pigeon could press to receive a food reward to reinforce a behavior. He manipulated the behavior with stimuli such as lights, tones and electrical shocks to study the rate, probability and force of a repeatable response. Skinner's detailed study of animal behavior set the stage for later studies on animal learning. Using computers with modern-day Skinner's boxes, scientists can predict animal behavior with a high degree of probability.

Skinner applied his scientific discoveries regarding behavior to a wide range of social and political problems. He was an ardent inventor who developed a missile guidance system in WWII using pigeons in the nose cone to locate a target ship, a baby crib (temperature and humidity controlled) that allowed the child to move about in a safe environment and a teaching machine that could help children learn to read using positive reinforcement. In his book *The Technology of Teaching,* he noted that teachers must understand the scientific underpinning of learning if they are to be successful [49]. He warned against using aversive techniques and advised the frequent use of positive reinforcement. He wrote a letter to the California senate that eventually lead to a ban on spanking children in schools. In his book *Walden Two*, Skinner described a fictional community in the 1940s United States whose citizens were happy and productive because they used scientific social planning and operant conditioning in raising their children [50]. Skinner emphasized the importance of friendship, health and art and of a balance between work and leisure to have a happy life. He wrote of his hope that improved understanding of the human science of behavioral control would help solve some of the unforeseen problems of rapid technological advancement. The work of Skinner and other behaviorists around the world led to the development of behavioral therapy which is still a major part of the management of patients with stress-related symptoms (see Chap. 10).

Skinner's view that voluntary behavior was primarily reflexive in origin based on external stimuli was revolutionary at the time but it failed to address a key feature of human behavior – much of our behavior is controlled by plans for the future not just the present or the past. Beliefs and expectations molded by our parents and society strongly influence these plans. Furthermore, the range of human behavior is so varied and complex that it would be difficult if not impossible to explain it on the basis of environmental stimuli alone. Although a discussion of the organization of higher forms of human consciousness, including awareness of self, are beyond the scope of this book, I address the role of beliefs and expectations on sickness behavior in the next chapter.

In Brief

The limbic system, the emotional center of the brain, is formed by a large arc of the medial brain connected to the hypothalamus, the neuroendocrine center of the brain located at the top of the brainstem. Nerve impulses arriving at the hypothalamus trigger the release of adrenaline from the adrenal medulla and corticosteroids from the adrenal cortex. These hormones produce a variety of bodily symptoms and contribute to the changes in brain chemistry and connectivity associated with chronic stress. Neuroplasticity in the brain, particularly in the hippocampus of the limbic system, is critical for learning and storage of new information and chronic stress alters neuroplasticity by decreasing nerve growth factors and activating the immune system. Central sensitization is a type of neuroplasticity whereby repetitive incoming sensory signals are magnified by increased excitatory transmission and/or decreased inhibitory transmission. Another component of the limbic system, the amygdala is important for fear conditioning. Stress-related incoming signals to the amygdala can lead to hypersensitization of a subgroup of excitatory neurons that are normally kept in check by inhibitory feedback from neurons in the prefrontal cortex, a part of the cortex critical for planning and problem solving. An imbalance between excitation and inhibition in these neurons in the amygdala can lead to a state of chronic fear and anxiety. Human behavior, including sick behavior, is a learned response dependent on neuroplasticity and is subject to reward and punishment reinforcement just like other forms of learning.

References

1. Levone BR, Cryan JF, O'Leary OF. Role of adult hippocampal neurogenesis in stress resilience. Neurobiol Stress. 2015;1:147e155.
2. Elliott GR, Eisdorfer C. Stress and human health. New York: Springer; 1982.
3. Segerstrom SC, Miller GE. Psychological stress and the human immune system: a meta-analytic study of 30 years of inquiry. Psychol Bull. 2004;130:601–30.
4. Liu LY, Coe CL, Swenson CA, et al. School examination enhances airway inflammation to antigen challenge. Am J Respir Crit Care Med. 2002;165:1062–7.
5. Mohd RS. Life event, stress and illness. Malays J Med Sci. 2008;15:9–18.
6. Rajendran K, Rao VN, Reddy MV. A profile of stressful life events among industrial neurotics and normal. NIMHANS J. 1996;14:127–32.
7. Cannon WB. Bodily changes in pain, hunger, fear and rage: an account of recent researches into the function of emotional excitement. New York: Appleton; 1915.
8. Papez JW. A proposed mechanism of emotion. Arch Neurol Psychiatr. 1937;38:725–43.
9. Lanska DJ. The Klüver-Bucy syndrome. Front Neurol Neurosci. 2018;41:41–77.
10. Selye H. Stress and psychiatry. Am J Psychiatry. 1956;113:423–7.
11. Pavlov IP. Conditioned reflexes. An investigation of the physiological activity of the cerebral cortex (translated by Anrep GV). London: Oxford University Press; 1927.
12. Cajal SR. The Croonian lecture: the fine structure of the nervous system. Proc R Soc Lond. 1894;Ser B55:444–67.
13. Milner OM, Milner B. Donald Olding Hebb: 22 July 1904-20 August 1985. Biogr Mem Fellows R Soc. 1996;42:193–204.
14. Obituary: Donald Olding Hebb (1904–1985) TINS, August 1986. p. 384.
15. Hebb DO. The organization of behavior. New York: Wiley; 1949.
16. Kandel ER. In search of memory. New York: WW Norton & Co; 2006.
17. Kempermann G, Gage FH, Aigner L, et al. Human adult neurogenesis: evidence and remaining questions. Cell Stem Cell. 2018;23:25–30.
18. Deppermann S, Storchak H, Fallgatter AJ, Ehlis AC. Stress-induced neuroplasticity: (Mal) adaptation to adverse life events in patients with PTSD – a critical overview. Neuroscience. 2014;283:166–77.
19. Levone BR, Cryan JF, O'Leary OF. Role of adult hippocampal neurogenesis in stress resilience. Neurobiology. 2015;1:147–55.
20. Micheli L, Ceccarelli M, D'Andrea G, Tirone F. Depression and adult neurogenesis: positive effects of the antidepressant fluoxetine and physical exercise. Brain Res Bull. 2018;143:181–93.
21. Notaras M, van den Buuse M. Neurobiology of BDNF in fear memory, sensitivity to stress, and stress-related disorders. Mol Psychiatry. 2020. Epub Jan 3.
22. Park DJ, Lee SS. New insights into the genetics of fibromyalgia. Korean J Intern Med. 2017;32:984–95.
23. Notaras M, van den Buuse M. Brain-derived neurotrophic factor (BDNF): novel insights into regulation and genetic variation. Neuroscientist. 2019;25:434–54.
24. Miller AH, Maletic V, Raison CL. Inflammation and its discontents: the role of cytokines in the pathophysiology of major depression. Biol Psychiatry. 2009;65:732–41.
25. Raison CL, Capuron L, Miller AH. Cytokines sing the blues: inflammation and the pathogenesis of depression. Trends Immunol. 2006;27:24–31.
26. Koo JW, Duman RS. Evidence for IL-1 receptor blockade as a therapeutic strategy for the treatment of depression. Curr Opin Investig Drugs. 2009;10:664–71.
27. Neugebauer V. Amygdala pain mechanisms. Handb Exp Pharmacol. 2015;227:261–84.
28. Baloh RW. Sciatica and chronic pain: past present and future. Cham: Springer; 2019. p. 71–85.
29. Basbaum AI, Fields HL. Endogenous pain control: brainstem spinal pathways and endorphin circuitry. Ann Rev Neurosci. 1984;7:309–38.
30. Beecher HK. Pain in men wounded in battle. Ann Surg. 1946;123:96–105.

31. Popoli M, Yan Z, McEwen B, Sanacora G. The stressed synapse: the impact of stress and glu-cocorticoids on glutamate transmission. Nat Rev Neurosci. 2013;13:22–37.
32. McEwen BS. Stress and hippocampal plasticity. Ann Rev Neurosci. 1999;22:105–22.
33. Liston C, Miller MM, Goldwater DS, Radley JJ, Rocher AB, Hof PR, et al. Stress-induced alterations in prefrontal cortical dendritic morphology predict selective impairments in percep-tual attentional set-shifting. J Neurosci. 2006;26:7870–4.
34. Cerqueira JJ, Mailliet F, Almeida OF, et al. The prefrontal cortex as a key target of the mal-adaptive response to stress. J Neurosci. 2007;27:2781–7.
35. Sanacora G, Zarate CA, Krystal JH, Manji HK. Targeting the glutamatergic system to develop novel, improved therapeutics for mood disorders. Nat Rev Drug Discov. 2008;7:426–37.
36. Giordano R, Pellegrino M, Picu A, et al. Neuroregulation of the hypothalamus-pituitary-adrenal (HPA) axis in humans: effects of GABA-, mineralocorticoid-, and GH-secretagogue-receptor modulation. Sci World J. 2006;6:1–11.
37. Gonda X, Petschner P, Eszlari N, et al. Effects of different stressors are modulated by different neurobiological systems: the role of GABA-A versus CB1 receeptor gene variants in anxiety and depression. Front Cell Neurosci. 2019;13:138.
38. Samuels ER, Szabadi E. Functional neuroanatomy of the noradrenergic locus coeruleus: its roles in the regulation of arousal and autonomic function. Part I: principles of functional orga-nization. Curr Neuropharmacol. 2008;6:235–53.
39. Yalcin I, Barrot M. The anxiodepressive comorbidity in chronic pain. Curr Opin Anaesthesiol. 2014;27:520–7.
40. Olds J, Milner P. Positive reinforcement produced by electrical stimulation of septal area and other regions of rat brain. J Comp Physiol Psychol. 1954;47:419–27.
41. Denk F, McMahon SB, Tracey I. Pain vulnerability: a neurobiological perspective. Nat Neurosci. 2014;17(2):192–200.
42. Leknes S, Tracey I. A common neurobiology for pain and pleasure. Nat Rev Neurosci. 2008;9:314–20.
43. Leknes S, Berna C, Lee MC, et al. The importance of context: when relative relief renders pain pleasant. Pain. 2013;154:402–10.
44. Patel S, Hillard CJ. Adaptations in endocannabinoid signaling in response to repeated homo-typic stress: a novel mechanism for stress habituation. Eur J Neurosci. 2008;27:2821–9.
45. Gorzalka BB, Hill MN, Hillard CJ. Regulation of endocannabinoid signaling by stress: impli-cations for stress-related affective disorders. Neurosci Biobehav Rev. 2008;32:11523–160.
46. Christensen R, Kristensen PK, Bartels EM, et al. Efficacy and safety of the weight-loss drug rimonabant: a meta analysis of randomized trials. Lancet. 2007;371:558.
47. Skinner BF. About behaviorism. New York: Random House; 1974. p. 20.
48. Skinner BF. Behavior of organisms. New York: Appleton-Century-Crofts; 1938.
49. Skinner BF. The technology of teaching. New York: Appleton-Century-Crofts; 1968.
50. Altus DE. Skinner's utopian vision: behind and beyond Walden Two. Behav Anal. 2009;32:319–35.

Psychosocial Mechanisms of Psychosomatic Symptoms

6

Learning that a symptom may be more noteworthy or medically significant amplifies it.

Arthur J. Barsky [1]

Everyone has heard of a placebo. Some would argue that placebos are better than most drugs currently available. When used in treatment trials for new drugs, placebo response rates are as high as 40%. By comparison, some of the best drugs have response rates of 60–70%. The placebo effect is a direct result of the person's expectation that the treatment will help. Functional MRI studies show activation (increase nerve firing) in the motivational/reward network and the descending pain modulatory system (DPMS) (see Chap. 5), with placebos and high placebo responders showing more activity in these areas than low responders [2]. Placebo effects are clearly influenced by the enthusiasm and expectations of the physician administering the treatment or by the surgeon performing an operation. A group of Swiss physicians suggested that the term "Curabo effect" be used to explain the fact that patients undergoing low back surgery without a clear indication had a better outcome if the surgeon was overly optimistic than if the surgeon was not optimistic [3].

Positive expectations are helpful, but negative expectations can be harmful. The so-called "nocebo effect," in which a person expects a negative outcome, is less well known but is critically important for understanding psychosomatic symptoms. Not surprisingly, activity in the motivational/reward network and the DPMS show the reverse effect on functional MRI (decreased firing) with the nocebo effect compared to the placebo effect [4]. Just as a patient is more likely to obtain benefit from a fake pill if they have positive expectations, they are more likely to have side effects from a fake pill if they have negative expectations. Providing a detailed description of possible side effects increases the risk of developing side effects. Remarkably, between 5% and 25% of patients in medical trials who are receiving a placebo drop out of the study because of perceived side effects. For example, in a treatment trial of fibromyalgia, 11% of patients taking a placebo dropped out of the study owing to the side effects of dizziness and nausea. People, of course, were told of these symptoms as possible side effects of the real drug used in the study. The nocebo effect occurs whether people receive a placebo or a real drug as long as they are told of the potential side effects. In other words, some of the side effects reported by patients receiving any drug are due to the nocebo effect. In a trial of the drug finasteride, commonly used for treating prostate enlargement and baldness in men, half of the participants were warned that the medication could cause erectile dysfunction, while the other half were not told about this possible side effect. Of those told about the potential side effect, 44% of those receiving finasteride reported experiencing erectile dysfunction, whereas only 15% of those not told about the potential side effect reported erectile dysfunction [5]. Health professionals obviously face an ethical dilemma when faced with the placebo and nocebo effects. Should they be overly optimistic about treatments and hide potential side effects from the patient? Aside from the fact that this would be illegal and would place the health professionals at risk of a law suit, it is also unethical. However, physicians can be trained to carefully balance the good and bad effects of treatments by providing accurate information but with reassurance and avoiding excessive negativity.

Health professionals often face a similar dilemma when dealing with a probable outbreak of psychosomatic illness. If a student or worker in an enclosed environment complains that they became sick after noticing a foul smell or a strange sound, should other students and workers be told about the incident and be on the alert should they smell the odor or hear the sound [6]? After all, there could be a dangerous toxin being released into the environment. In these instances, the picture is complicated by social and mass media that thrive on sensational stories. As when dealing with a single patient, health professional must strike a balance between providing truthful information and reassurance while at the same time combatting negative rumors.

Beliefs and expectations strongly influence the perception of somatic symptoms and response to treatments. If you believe a treatment will work, it likely will be effective (the placebo effect), whereas if you believe it won't work, it likely won't (the nocebo effect). If you expect to get a symptom, you probably will get the symptom. As discussed in Chap. 5, positive and negative expectations alter brain function, leading to changes in the body's biological systems, including the endocrine, cardiovascular and immune systems. Scientists have performed numerous controlled studies demonstrating the power of these effects. For example, belief that a nutrient is beneficial can improve the body's physiological response to the nutrient [7], and the health effects of exercise can be improved if a person believes that exercise will help [8]. The powerful effects of expectation on drug efficacy were demonstrated by giving participants a standard dose of an opioid drug before exposing them to a painful heat stimulus [9]. Those who were given no expectations had a moderate reduction in pain, whereas those who were told the drug would have a strong effect on pain had twice the pain relief as those with no expectations and those who were told the drug could have negative effects had no pain relief. People who believe that stress can be detrimental to their health have higher levels of stress hormones than people who believe that stress can enhance their health. In a provocative study of nearly 30,000 people in which the level of stress was controlled for, those who believed stress was harmful were much more likely to die prematurely than those who believed stress was not harmful [10].

How Can Beliefs and Expectations Change Brain Function?

Unlike digital computers, in which new information is stored in available space on a memory chip and the information is retrieved by simply reading the information back from the memory chip, the brain stores information by modifying existing circuits and synapses (as described in Chap. 5) that already contain stored information, including information about beliefs and expectations. When one attempts to retrieve the information, it is altered by prior experiences including beliefs and expectations. One's mindset has a major influence on how we store and retrieve information and how we react to somatic symptoms. If we expect pain to be relieved, connections between pain centers and the endogenous opioid system (e.g., the DPMS discussed in Chap. 5) are reinforced and pain signals are shut off on entering the spinal cord. On the other hand, if we expect pain to get worse, we focus on the pain, and pain circuits are reinforced, leading to central sensitization to pain. The same central sensitization mechanism (neuronal circuit enhancement) can occur with other somatic symptoms simply by focusing one's attention on the symptoms.

But how does the brain decide what information to focus on and what information to ignore? Keeping with the analogy of a digital computer – where is the central processor, the part of the brain that decides on what information to retrieve and in what order? The simple answer is that we don't know, but clearly it is not a highly localized brain center such as the one proposed by Descarte (see Chap. 2), where all information is constantly monitored and "strings" pulled to control appropriate responses. The central processor is almost certainly a distributed property of multiple brain regions and their interconnecting pathways. Information is stored within these pathways just as it is stored in all other brain pathways, by modifying existing circuits and synapses. The field of cognitive psychology focuses on the brain mechanisms that control thoughts and actions and thereby shape consciousness. Models of brain hierarchy have been proposed to explain somatization based on how the brain selects information for further processing and decides on appropriate action [11, 12]. A key component of these models is an "attentional system," neuronal circuits that use existing knowledge to identify relevant information to attend to for priority processing. A great deal of complex processing of information occurs prior to arrival at the attentional system, and the attentional system uses current information from sensory, perceptual and memory systems to control behavior and to inform conscious awareness. Keep in mind that these models consist of "black boxes" that represent brain mechanisms that have yet to be characterized at the cellular level, but the models are testable as new information is identified, and they provide a working model to understand how psychosomatic symptoms might arise.

British psychologist Richard Brown proposed a model to explain psychosomatic symptoms in which he divided the attentional system into two parts, a primary system that performs operations perceived as effortless and self-evident and a secondary system that performs operations perceived as effortful and deliberate, associated with self-awareness [13]. This model allows for a dissociation between one's experience and what is really happening so that what people believe or want to believe can take precedence over what their sensory systems are telling them is actually happening. In the model, the primary attentional system is automatically activated when information from the perceptual or memory systems reaches a threshold level of activation. Psychosomatic symptoms can arise when the primary attentional system selects inappropriate information from chronically activated stored information. Brown described what he called "rogue representations," defined as inappropriate information selected by the primary attentional system that can serve as a template for the development of psychosomatic symptoms. The inappropriate information could come from any source, including memories of prior illness in oneself or others. Seeing others experiencing symptoms can activate neuronal circuits that are identical to those activated when you experience symptoms yourself. Rogue representations can develop from a variety of other types of stored information, including information obtained from friends, doctors, the media, the internet and sociocultural beliefs. Constantly attending to a symptom, such as frequently checking to see if it is still there, amplifies the symptom so that the selection threshold is lowered and less activation is required for the symptom to be selected by the attentional system, a process similar to central hypersensitivity discussed in Chap. 5. Although everyone is potentially susceptible to developing rogue representations, certain people are more susceptible based on genetic, personality, and environmental factors.

Doctor-Patient Relationship and Psychosomatic Symptoms

As noted on numerous occasions throughout this book, the doctor -patient relationship plays a critical role in the process of symptom amplification. When the doctor attributes a symptom to a new and potentially serious disease, the patient naturally becomes more focused and attentive toward the symptom, which makes it more intense and distressing [1]. This process, often called misattribution, causes the patient to search for additional symptoms to corroborate the new diagnosis, leading to amplification of everyday nonspecific symptoms previously thought to be insignificant. This vicious cycle of symptom amplification further initiates fear and anxiety, which can trigger a range of somatic symptoms on its own. The result can be the development of a defined symptom complex such as fibromyalgia or chronic fatigue syndrome. On the other hand, if early in the process the physician recognizes that the symptoms are not the manifestation of a serious disease and provides the patient with reassurance that they are not due to a serious life-threatening illness, the symptoms become less significant and may eventually resolve.

Research shows that it is not just the doctor's words that matter [1]. The doctor's demeanor, appearance and understanding all make a difference. An empathetic doctor can decrease patient anxiety, improve the patient's mood and alleviate worry and concerns, all of which improve outcomes. Furthermore, if patients perceive the doctor as empathetic and understanding, they are less likely to demand unnecessary tests and treatments that can lead to symptom attribution and amplification. This physician placebo effect also holds for prescribed medications where studies show that physician presentation, labeling, price, and even color of the pill can influence the patient's response [14]. These physician effects are not just important for outcome in patients with psychogenic illness but also for a range of organic disorders, including cancer. Even the severity and duration of a common cold can be altered by the patient's perception of the physician's empathy [15].

The Power of the Placebo

Placebos are all about expectations and beliefs. What you expect and what you believe are critically important in determining your health. Whether it's the outcome of a drug treatment, surgery, cognitive behavioral therapy, acupuncture or mindfulness therapy, all are highly influenced by the placebo effect. Much of the clinical work on placebos has been done in drug trials where placebos are routinely used. It wasn't until the latter half of the twentieth century that researchers realized the importance of the placebo effect, however. In 1955, the American anesthesiologist Henry Beecher (mentioned in Chap. 4 for his observation that many soldiers did not complain of pain despite serious wounds) wrote an article in the Journal of the American Medical Association entitled "The Powerful Placebo," warning researchers that studies of new drugs must contain a placebo in order to properly evaluate the true drug effect [16]. In the twenty-first century, drug treatment trials are not considered valid unless the drug effect is compared with the placebo effect.

As the number of drug trials increased, it became apparent that participants often receive clues as to whether or not they are receiving the active drug. Typically, physicians conducting the studies are "blinded" as to who is receiving the active drug but participants can still get cues regarding who is receiving the active drug based on the taste and side effects. Studies show that the placebo effect is greater if placebo pills are large and have a bitter taste compared to small inert sugar pills [17]. Adding something to the placebo pill that produces a noticeable side effect can also enhance the effectiveness. It follows that all drugs have a placebo effect in addition to any true drug effect. Drug companies have learned to optimize the placebo effect of new drugs by choosing brand names that suggest potency. For example, they have found that using the letters X and Z in the name seems to connote efficacy and that capsules are perceived as more powerful than tablets [18]. How large is the placebo effect versus the true drug effect for commonly used drugs? Although the data are not always available, the placebo component is probably at least 50% of the total effect for most commonly used drugs. For example, the commonly used nonsteroidal anti-inflammatory drugs (NSAIDs such as ibuprofen and naproxen) are only half as effective if they are given without the patient's knowledge compared to when they are given with the patient's understanding that they are receiving a pain pill [19]. Analysis of the massive data collected by the US Food and Drug Administration (FDA) on clinical trials of antidepressant drugs found that overall the efficacy of placebos was 65% of the efficacy of the antidepressant drugs [20]. However, even this number is probably an underestimation of the placebo effect. In the few studies of antidepressant drugs in which placebos were used that produced noticeable side effects, there was no significant difference in the efficacy of the drug versus placebo [21]. This sobering observation suggests that we may be spending billions of dollars a year on medications for depression with significant side effects that are no better than placebos.

Placebo effects are part of all treatments, not just drug treatments. In fact, the placebo effect may be even greater for treatments involving "the laying on of hands" such as surgery, physical therapy, acupuncture and chiropractor manipulations. It is very difficult to have a true placebo in clinical trails with these types of interventions since it is difficult, if not impossible, to blind the surgeon or therapist performing the procedures, and sham procedures are often apparent to the participants. Although relatively few placebo-controlled treatment trials of surgical procedures have been performed (for obvious ethical reasons), those that have been conducted have shown a dramatic placebo effect. In a review of published studies in 2014, in slightly more than 50% of studies the sham procedure produced results equal to that of the actual surgical procedure [22]. In studies where there is a nonintervention control group, sham surgery produces significantly improved outcomes compared to no treatment. Numerous placebo trials have been attempted to evaluate the effectiveness of physical therapy, acupuncture and chiropractic manipulations, but detailed analysis of these studies by impartial observers found that the studies are impossible to interpret because of the difficulties in conducting true placebo sham procedures. In summary, there is no scientifically sound evidence that these procedures are any better than placebo [23].

How do we explain the placebo effect? Much of our understanding of the mechanisms of placebos comes from the study of placebos for pain control. As discussed in Chap. 5, expectation of a placebo effect activates brain pain control systems such as the endogenous opioid system and the motivation/reward system. There is also a major role for learning with the placebo response. People can be taught to increase their response to placebos just as Pavlov's dogs were conditioned to increase salivation when hearing a bell ring. For example, if patients are repeatedly exposed to a moderately painful stimulus in the first phase of a study and then in the second phase are given a placebo before being exposed to a lesser painful stimulus that was reduced without their knowledge, they associate the placebo with pain relief [24]. Later, they have an enhanced placebo response when exposed to the moderate painful stimulus due to "learning" (increased connectivity) within brain pain control pathways. This enhanced placebo response can cross over to other drugs so that they are better placebo responders in general. Similarly, if someone sees other people receiving effective pain relief from a medication, they are more likely to receive pain relief from the same medication [25]. This type of observational learning likely occurs in clinics and hospitals where patients can talk with other patients who have received similar medications. These learning effects are not confined to just pain medications but are relevant to a wide range of medications, even including immunosuppressive drugs used for renal transplant patients [26].

Researchers who perform clinical trials on new drugs have long been aware that the placebo response is very variable. Some people are clearly better placebo responders than others. Could it be that some people are conditioned to respond to placebos? Could there be a genetic basis for the placebo response? The answer to both of these questions is yes, although research into the neurobiology and genetics of the placebo response is in its infancy. One disquieting possibility in the age of universal placebo-controlled treatment trials is that the reason drugs that are found to be significantly better than placebo in these trials is due to improvement in the placebo response rather than improvement in the underlying disorder [27]. Naturally, drug researchers and pharmaceutical companies would dismiss this possibility and argue that they choose and develop drugs based on the effect they have on the presumed disease mechanisms. But the idea of drugs improving the placebo response is not farfetched and based on the way treatment trials are conducted, increasing the placebo effect cannot be distinguished from decreasing the disease effect. Interestingly, preliminary studies of variations in genes (polymorphisms) identified as increasing the response to placebos found that the affected genes code for proteins that are the target of many widely used drugs, including common drugs for treating pain, anxiety and depression. Of 54 genes identified as altering the placebo response in clinical drug trials, 40 are known drug targets [27]. Once these genetic susceptibility variants have been replicated in future studies, they will have to be controlled for so that placebo susceptibility is equally divided between the drug and placebo arms of a study.

Placebo's Evil Twin, Nocebo

Although the importance of the placebo effect on medical treatments is widely recognized by medical researchers and the general public, the importance of the nocebo effect is relatively unknown. As we will see, however, understanding the mechanism of the nocebo effect is critical to understanding the mechanism of psychosomatic symptoms. On analysis of placebo-controlled clinical drug trials, about a quarter of patients receiving placebo report side effects and about three quarters of side effects reported by patients receiving active drugs are likely not do to the drug effect but rather due to the nocebo effect [17]. Supporting this observation, if participants (receiving placebo or active drug) are specifically asked about certain side effects they are much more likely to report having the side effects. Two remarkable examples of the importance of the nocebo effect in public health are the controversies over side effects of the commonly used statin drugs and the role of sensitivity to gluten in causing a wide range of medical symptoms.

Statins and Muscle Pain and Weakness

One could reasonably argue that statins (e.g., atorvastatin, lovastatin, simvastatin and pravastatin) have had the most significant impact on public health of any class of drugs introduced in the twentieth century. By lowering "bad lipids," these drugs decrease the risk of heart attacks and stroke, two of the main causes of death in modern society. Shortly after these drugs became widely used, however, patients began reporting muscle pain, soreness and weakness, causing them to stop taking the drugs and even dampening physician's enthusiasm for prescribing the drugs. These symptoms were widely reported by the media and alarmed patients confronted their doctors about the risk of continuing these "dangerous" medications. This occurred even though analysis of several large placebo-controlled treatment trials did not show a significant difference in muscle symptoms in the placebo- and drug-treated patients [28, 29]. Even more important, large studies in Denmark and England found that negative news stories about statins in the media correlated with early discontinuation of statins, which in turn lead to an increase in deaths from heart attacks [30, 31]. Although rarely patients do develop muscle damage from statins, the vast majority of muscle symptoms in patients taking statins can be explained by the nocebo effect and the risk/benefit ratio for statins is one of the lowest for any of the commonly used drugs.

Glutens and Celiac Disease

Gluten is a protein in a variety of grains, including wheat, rye and barley. It gives the flour from these grains a glue-like consistency, which is useful in making bread and other dough products. Between a half to one percent of the population develop antibodies directed at gluten, causing an autoimmune disease called celiac disease, which is manifested by inflammation of the gut and a variety of gastrointestinal and systemic symptoms. By contrast, from 5% to 10% of the population believe they are intolerant to gluten and attribute a wide range of symptoms from abdominal discomfort and bloating to fatigue and headache to ingesting gluten. However, these people do not have antibodies associated with celiac disease or structural changes in the gut. Placebo-controlled gluten-exposure trials have failed to show that gluten-sensitive people who do not have celiac disease have more symptoms with gluten than with placebo and gluten-sensitive people do not develop symptoms when given gluten protein without their knowledge [32]. Despite the evidence that gluten sensitivity is due to negative expectations, the nocebo effect, a large industry has developed to produce gluten-free foods, and perceived gluten sensitivity is a major inconvenience to affected people and their families.

Expectations and Beliefs

People's expectations and beliefs play a major role in defining the magnitude of the nocebo response. In placebo-controlled treatment trials, if people are told about a possible side effect, they are much more likely to develop the side effect whether they receive a placebo or the actual medication. The types of side effects attributed to placebo medications are largely determined by the common side effects of the active drug in the trial, the side effects typically listed on the informed consent form for the trial [33]. If people enter a drug trial with the preconceived notion that they are very sensitive to medications, they are much more likely to have side effects whether they receive the active drug or a placebo [34]. Similarly, people with perceived sensitivity to drugs are more likely to develop symptoms after receiving travel vaccines, and parents who believe that vaccines can impair their child's health are more likely to report side effects in their children after vaccines. People who believe that they are very sensitive to medications are much more likely to go on the internet and read about possible side effects, further increasing the likelihood of developing the side effects. Those who believe brand-name drugs are better than generic drugs are more likely to develop side effects from a generic drug, even if the generic drug was switched to a brand-name drug without their knowledge [35]. If a person develops side effects from a specific drug, the same side effects can continue after the drug is replaced by a placebo, and people with drug reactions in the past are much more likely to develop side effects from new, unrelated drugs. Finally, seeing other people experiencing side effects from a medication, whether in person or on television, can increase the likelihood of the observer developing side effects from the medication [36].

As with the placebo response, conditioned learning can occur with the nocebo response. Just as Pavlov's dogs learned to associate food with the white coat of the research associates who fed them, cancer patients receiving chemotherapy can develop nausea just from the smell of the treatment room or upon seeing a known a white-coated clinic member [37]. A group of psychologists in Belgium developed an innovative laboratory model to study the effect of learning and expectancy on psychogenic symptoms and made several interesting observations [38]. They induced a variety of common symptoms, including a smothering sensation, chest tightness, sweating, palpitations, lump in the throat, headache, dizziness and anxiety, by having test subjects inhale air enriched with 7.5% carbon dioxide for 2 min. Since carbon dioxide has no smell or taste, it could be administered without discomfort, and symptoms reliably began about 20 s after inhalation and stopped quickly after the trial. For the learning trials, they added an odor to the carbon dioxide–enriched air for three trials and then presented the odor with regular air and monitored physiological changes and symptom intensity. Subjects regularly learned to associate the odor with the symptoms and developed symptoms after just the odor without enriched carbon dioxide. In addition to pungent odors, they found that negative thoughts such as imagining being trapped in an enclosed space while experiencing the smothering sensation induced by the carbon dioxide led to development of the same symptoms after just the thought of being in an elevator without receiving carbon dioxide. Interestingly, the development of symptoms only occurred if they used a foul-smelling odor and not with a pleasant or neutral odor and with negative thoughts and not with neutral or positive thoughts. These learning effects were most pronounced in subjects who scored high on negativity scales and who had a history of experiencing psychosomatic symptoms. The results clearly illustrate how human learning is affected by expectations, particularly negative expectations, and how symptoms that were initially associated with abnormal physiology may later be triggered by a thought or environmental cue.

Hyperventilation Syndrome

The results of these studies with inhaled carbon dioxide also provide potentially new insights into understanding the controversial "hyperventilation syndrome." Not only increasing but also decreasing the level of carbon dioxide in the blood can cause somatic symptoms. When I trained in neurology in the 1970s, the hyperventilation syndrome was touted as the prototypical psychogenic syndrome with a clear physiological explanation. When patients become anxious, particularly when having a panic attack, they hyperventilate, lowering the carbon dioxide pressure in the blood, which in turn causes constriction of the smooth muscles in the walls of cerebral blood vessels, so-called vasoconstriction. Blood carbon dioxide concentration is a well-known regulator of brain blood flow. The decreased brain blood flow due to low carbon dioxide levels caused a variety of symptoms, including headache, dizziness, disorientation, impaired concentration, and even fainting. It is still not uncommon to see people in public places breathing into paper bags, the recommended treatment for hyperventilation syndrome. By breathing into the bag, they rebreathe exhaled carbon dioxide, which increases blood carbon dioxide concentration. But when studies were performed on patients with hyperventilation syndrome first in the laboratory and then during real life episodes in the mid-1990s, researchers found a poor correlation between symptoms and blood carbon dioxide concentration [39, 40]. Although low blood carbon dioxide was found in occasional patients, the symptoms seemed to correlate much better with anxiety levels than with carbon dioxide concentration. In many cases, they could find no obvious cause for the symptoms. These observations led researchers to question the scientific validity of the concept of hyperventilation syndrome and recommended discontinuing its use as a clinical diagnosis. But what if hyperventilation and low blood carbon dioxide levels caused symptoms during initial "learning episodes" and subsequent episodes were triggered by environmental or thought cues that became conditioned stimuli for the symptoms? This hypothesis that symptoms induced by abnormal physiology or even pathology can be learned and environmental and thought cues associated with the symptoms during the learning process later become conditional stimuli for the symptoms, can explain many of the symptoms of a variety of psychosomatic disorders and is testable in research settings. Furthermore, the hypothesis is consistent with how the brain learns new information as discussed in Chap. 5.

Idiopathic Environmental Intolerance and the Nocebo Effect

Idiopathic environmental intolerance refers to a group of poorly understood medical conditions in which a wide variety of somatic symptoms occur in response to environmental exposures: chemicals, electromagnetic fields, infrasound and even the interior of certain buildings [41]. No clear link with organ damage or dysfunction has been established with any of these disorders, and there is a general consensus that the symptoms are psychosomatic in origin overlapping the symptoms of fibromyalgia, chronic fatigue syndrome and Gulf War syndrome. There is strong evidence that expectancy and nocebo mechanisms are involved in producing the symptoms, and conditioned learning, as described in the prior section, can explain how symptoms initially come about and become linked to specific environmental cues.

Multiple chemical sensitivity develops from perceived exposure to low levels of commonly used chemicals, particularly those with an odor [42]. Although most people with multiple chemical sensitivity perceive that they are sensitive to many environmental chemicals, some develop symptoms after a single chemical exposure such as occurs when in the vicinity of a perceived terrorist chemical attack or chemical spill. Symptoms include headache, dizziness, fatigue, difficulties concentrating, brain fog, memory impairment and shortness of breath and in more than half of patients the symptoms are chronic and disabling [43]. All researchers agree that the prevalence of multiple chemical sensitivity is rapidly increasing in modern societies; a population-based study of Australian adults found that 6.5% reported a medical diagnosis of multiple chemical sensitivity and 19% reported having adverse reactions to multiple chemicals [44]. The female/male ratio of multiple chemical sensitivity is about 3/1. Common chemical triggers include cleaning products, tobacco smoke, perfume and vehicle fumes, but studies have not found a clear association between the perceived chemical pollutants and specific symptoms. Sufferers spend large sums of money changing household cleaning and personal hygiene products and purchasing air and water filters, and many frequently change residences and jobs. Blinded clinical provocation trials using fake chemicals (placebos) show that people with multiple chemical sensitivity develop the same symptoms whether exposed to real or fake chemicals [45]. There is no evidence for allergy or other toxic tissue damage from the chemical exposure. As with other nocebo effects, an individual's expectations and beliefs play a major role in the development of symptoms associated with multiple chemical sensitivity syndrome. Negative expectations and beliefs ("My body is very sensitive to chemicals") are amplified by the mass media and health professionals and reinforced by friends and family with similar beliefs.

The Belgium Coca-Cola Fiasco

Large outbreaks of mass psychogenic illness have also been attributed to perceived chemical exposure. One of the most dramatic such episodes began in Bornem, Belgium in 1999 when several school children became sick after drinking Coca-Cola that they reported had a foul odor [46]. After sensational stories appeared on TV and in newspapers suggesting that Coca-Cola was poisoning young children, outbreaks occurred in several other schools in nearby cities, and adult citizens flooded the Belgium poison control hotline with reports of being sick after drinking Coca-Cola and other soft drinks. The main symptoms were headache, dizziness, nausea, difficulty catching breath, malaise, abdominal discomfort and trembling. Despite extensive laboratory testing, no evidence of a toxin could be found in the patients or the tainted Coca-Cola. As companies are instructed to do in these situations, the Coca-Cola Company apologized and suggested that there might have been a problem with the carbonation process since they found trace amounts of foul-smelling H_2S in a few of the bottles, even though the amount was too small to cause symptoms. As the outbreak spread through Belgium and to other European countries, Coca-Cola products were ordered removed from store shelves first in Belgium and then in France, Spain, Germany, Holland and Luxembourg, overall costing the giant soft drink company more than 300 million dollars. As the outbreak began to subside, an *ad hoc* working group commissioned by the Belgian Health Ministry reported that no notable chemical toxins had been found, despite extensive studies, and that the outbreaks most likely represented a case of mass psychogenic illness. The outbreak was triggered by odors associated with non-toxic amounts of chemicals and occurred in a background of a population stressed by a prior toxic scare. In May 1999, the Belgian media reported that chickens had been contaminated with dioxin, a highly toxic environmental pollutant. Chickens and eggs were recalled followed shortly by dairy and meat products. Making matters worse, although the contamination occurred in February, it was not made public until May 25th, when it was leaked to the press. The uproar was so great that the Minister of Health and the Minister of Agriculture were forced to resign just before general elections in June. The media questioned the safety of modern-day foods, and scientists emphasized that even minute amounts of chemicals could seriously affect one's health.

The controversial conclusion that the Coca-Cola outbreak was due to mass psychogenic illness was presented to the public in a television program and presented to the scientific community in a letter to a well-respected scientific journal [47]. Despite the expected immediate backlash from physicians and the lay public questioning the working group's conclusion, as time went on and no further cases were identified the public began to accept the conclusion. The ban on Coca-Cola products in Belgium was lifted in June of 1999, but the Belgium government didn't officially exonerate Coca-Cola products and accept the mass psychogenic illness hypothesis until March of 2000.

As with all cases of mass psychogenic illness, medical personal and the media played an important role in the course of events. First line responders and emergency room physicians were obviously concerned in the face of a possible mass poisoning, especially in children, and appropriately took the matter very seriously. The media picked up on these concerns and reported the Coca-Cola poisoning as fact. In retrospect, the apology from the Coca-Cola company may have inadvertently made matters worse. As it became obvious that none of the children were seriously ill and most of the children were rapidly recovering, reassurance was appropriate for both the children and their families. In this setting, there really was no downside to calm, reassuring behavior by physicians and the media. Physicians at the Poison Control Center were obviously convinced of a poisoning epidemic and may have unwittingly contributed to the spread by directing all callers to go to their physician or to a hospital. Making matters worse, a physician called the Poison Control Center to ask if there had been any reports of hemolysis from drinking Coca-Cola. Hemolysis is a rupture of red blood cells that can be a sign of serious poisoning. This prompted the staff to record hemolysis as a possible effect of drinking Coca-Cola; the Health Minister picked up on this and mentioned it at a press conference. Not long after, a hospital reported 10 cases of hemolysis after consumption of Coca-Cola, which was immediately broadcast by the media. The smoking gun of a poisoning had been identified. Later analysis by a team of expert hematologists, however, found no evidence for hemolysis and concluded that the report was due to a technical artifact. Finally, the media played their usual role in reinforcing anxiety and anger in the public. They made frequent comparisons between the dioxin and Coca-Cola crises in headlines and editorials and showed pictures of loads of dead animals being dumped alongside crates of soft drinks being trashed.

Electromagnetic Hypersensitivity

Another common type of idiopathic environmental intolerance is the electromagnetic hypersensitivity syndrome whereby people attribute symptoms to exposure to electromagnetic fields, such as those produced by mobile phones and their relay stations, electric power lines and even remote-control devices. When mobile phones first came into general use, there were dire predictions that the electromagnetic waves associated with mobile phones would increase the risk of brain cancer just as smoking increased the risk of lung cancer. But over time the rate of brain cancer remained flat, despite the universal use of mobile phones. People attribute a variety of ear and brain symptoms, including tinnitus, dizziness, headaches and concentration difficulties, to electromagnetic waves [48, 49], but there is no scientific evidence that electromagnetic fields associated with mobile phones or any other device can damage the ear or brain. Double-blind provocative studies have shown that people who claim they experience symptoms from exposure to electromagnetic fields are unable to detect the presence of electromagnetic fields and sham exposure to electromagnetic fields causes symptoms as frequently as real exposure [50, 51]. Studies that assess people's expectations prior to being exposed to sham or real electromagnetic fields show that the nocebo effect plays a key role in determining whether symptoms develop or not. If people expect to have symptoms, they are much more likely to have them.

Not surprisingly, the media plays an important role in people's expectations. Media warnings about the adverse effects of modern life may be self-fulfilling. In a study on the effects of exposure to sham electromagnetic fields conducted in London, 147 healthy people were randomly assigned to watch a television documentary about the health effects of electromagnetic fields or a control documentary on mobile phones that did not mention health or electromagnetic fields [52]. Participants were told, "This project will assess whether a new type of electromagnetic field, which will be used in future mobile phones and WiFi systems, can cause short term physical symptoms such as fatigue or headaches" [53]. After watching the documentaries, subjects were fitted with a headband and an attached antenna and told that the device was meant to bring the signal as close to them as possible.

They were then told that they would be exposed to the electromagnetic field for 15 min and that they should watch for any symptoms that might develop during the exposure. They could terminate exposure if the symptoms became too strong. Eighty-two of the 147 participants (54%) reported symptoms, which they attributed to the sham electromagnetic field exposure. Having watched the TV documentary suggesting adverse health effects significantly increased the likelihood of people having symptoms after the sham exposure compared to the control group. People with pre-existing anxiety were more likely to develop symptoms than those without anxiety. Men and women were equally affected. There was also a hint that watching the threatening documentary could have long-term effects, since the participants who had watched that documentary and attributed their symptoms to the sham exposure were significantly more likely to think they had increased sensitivity to electromagnetic fields than those who had symptoms but watched the control documentary. They would be more likely to attribute symptoms to electromagnetic field exposure in the future.

Infrasound Sensitivity

A relatively recent form of idiopathic environmental intolerance is infrasound sensitivity, in which people attribute a variety of ear and brain symptoms to low-frequency sound exposure [54]. The ear symptoms include dizziness, tinnitus, earache and hypersensitivity to sound, while brain symptoms include headache, concentration and memory problems and sleep disorders. Wind turbines for generating clean energy have been around for decades, yet concerns about health effects did not surface until the 1990s, when it was first reported that wind turbines emitted infrasound [55]. But unlike some other potential mysterious environmental threats, it was easy to measure the power of infrasound emitted by modern-day wind turbines, and it was found to be in the same low range (20–40 decibels) as standing several meters from the ocean or a fan. But this fact and numerous scientific studies showing no ill health effects of low-energy infrasound exposure did not deter advocates from trying to ban wind turbines from their communities [56]. One might reasonably question whether the real reason for the desire to ban the wind turbines was the appearance of these massive structures next to residential areas rather than the concern for ill health effects. In fact, concerns about wind farms are probably more due to visual appearance and beliefs than to the wind turbine noise itself [57]. Studies in the Netherlands found that people who benefited economically from wind farms either with monthly stipends or partial ownership were much less likely to be annoyed by the noise than those without an economic interest [58]. People with an economic interest in wind farms had the same awareness and sensitivity to sound as those without an economic interest, but they had a different attitude toward the noise. Seeing and hearing the wind turbines didn't seem to bother them.

Sick Building Syndrome

Sometimes medical symptoms are attributed to being in a specific indoor environment [59]. Although the term "sick building syndrome" was introduced by the World Health Organization and is still widely used, critics have appropriately pointed out that buildings do not become sick and that another term, such as "building-related environmental intolerance," would be more appropriate. There is obvious overlap with the other environmental intolerance syndromes since people often attribute their symptoms to odors or sounds in the building, and many people with sick building syndrome have comorbidity with other types of environmental intolerance and with functional somatic syndromes and mood disorders. Population studies in Sweden and Finland found a prevalence of self-reported sick building syndrome of 5% and 7%, respectively [60]. Importantly, the vast majority reported symptoms from being in a building where other occupants had no symptoms. Typically, symptoms become worse the longer the person stays in the building, and symptoms gradually subside once out of the building. Occasionally, a possible cause for the symptoms such as an odor from cleaning chemicals or sounds originating from the heating and cooling ducts has been reported, but as with other environmental sensitivity syndromes, these findings are more likely triggers for the symptoms rather than the cause. Most of the time, no likely cause is found despite extensive investigation. The majority of patients with sick building syndrome develop avoidance behavior that can strengthen conditioned fear responses and in the long-term increase illness behavior.

Overview of Idiopathic Environmental Intolerance Mechanisms

There is a general consensus that the nocebo effect is the underlying mechanism for symptoms in patients with idiopathic environmental intolerance. The nocebo effect is associated with a general negative affect, including one's mood and sense of self-worth, and with a negative expectation of threat from the surrounding environment. People with negative affect are more likely to focus and ruminate on routine body symptoms and to attribute the symptoms to an external source such as an environmental toxin [61]. Conditioned learning plays a role, whereby symptoms perceived to be triggered by environmental stimuli are repeatedly paired with environmental stimuli, leading to long-term potentiation of brain pathways storing the sensory perceptions of the symptoms (central sensitization). Based on Brown's model for psychosomatic symptoms described earlier in this chapter, the "attentional system" selects "rogue representations" based on negative perceptions of the self and the environment that serve as a template for the development of symptoms. The negative perceptions come from a variety of sources, including prior personal experiences and suggestions of friends, family and the media. By attending to the symptoms, the symptoms are amplified so that the selection threshold is lowered and less activation is required for conscious awareness. In other words, a classic vicious cycle develops. With this understanding of basic brain mechanisms associated with psychosomatic symptoms, we are ready to tackle the problem of people with the most common medically unexplained symptoms, pain, fatigue and dizziness.

In Brief

Beliefs and expectations play a pivotal role in the production of psychosomatic symptoms. The placebo effect (expecting the positive) and the nocebo effect (expecting the negative) not only influence the response to treatment but also the perception of illness. Doctors help mold beliefs and expectations. Attributing symptoms to a potentially serious disease can amplify everyday symptoms previously thought to be insignificant. Focus on a symptom reinforces brain pathways generating the symptom, a type of central sensitization. Learning to associate symptoms with environmental events, such as tastes and smells, or with negative thoughts, such as being stuck on an elevator, can lead to changes in brain connectivity so that these events and thoughts become reliable triggers for the symptoms. These brain mechanisms likely explain a wide variety of symptoms attributed to environmental exposures that affect a surprisingly large percentage of the general population.

References

1. Barsky AJ. The iatrogenic potential of the physician's words. JAMA. 2017;318:2425.
2. Seminowicz DA. Believe in your placebo. J Neurosci. 2006;26:4453–4.
3. Graz B, Wietlisbach V, Porchet F, Vader J-P. Prognosis or "curabo effect?" : physician prediction and patient outcome of surgery for low back pain and sciatica. Spine (Phila Pa 1976). 2005;30(12):1448–52.
4. Benedetti F, Lanotte M, Lopiano L, Colloca L. When words are painful: unraveling the mechanisms of the nocebo effect. Neuroscience. 2007;147:260–71.
5. Enck P, Ha W. Beware the nocebo effect. The New York Times, 2012 August 10.
6. Baloh RW, Bartholomew R. Havana syndrome: the real story behind the embassy mystery illness and modern-day hysteria. New York: Springer; 2020.
7. Crum AJ, Corbin WR, Brownell KD, Salovey P. Mind over milkshakes: mindsets, not just nutrients, determine ghrelin response. Health Psychol. 2011;30:424–9.
8. Crum AJ, Langer EJ. Mind-set matters: exercise and the placebo effect. Psychol Sci. 2007;18:165–71.
9. Bingel U, Wanigasekera V, Wiech K, et al. The effect of treatment expectation on drug efficacy: imaging the analgesic benefit of the opioid Remifentanil. Sci Transl Med. 2011;3:70ra14.
10. Keller A, Litzelman K, Wisk LE. Does the perception that stress affects health matter? The association with health and mortality. Health Psychol. 2012;31:677–84.
11. Kirmayer LJ, Taillefer S. Somatoform disorders. In: Turner SM, Hersen M, editors. Adult psychopathology and diagnosis. 3rd ed. New York: Wiley; 1997. p. 333–83.
12. Styles EA. The psychology of attention. Hove: Psychology Press; 1997.
13. Brown RJ. Psychological mechanisms of medically unexplained symptoms: an integrative conceptual model. Psychol Bull. 2004;130:793–812.
14. Crum AJ, Leibowitz KA, Verghese A. Making mindset matter. BMJ. 2017;356:j674.

15. Rakel DP, Hoeft TJ, Barrett BP, et al. Practitioner empathy and the duration of the common cold. Fam Med. 2009;41:494–501.
16. Beecher HK. The powerful placebo. JAMA. 1955;159:1602–6.
17. Petrie KJ, Rief W. Psychobiological mechanisms of placebo and nocebo effects: pathways to improve treatments and reduce side effects. Annu Rev Psychol. 2019;70:599–625.
18. Stepney R. A dose by any other name would not sell as sweet. BMJ. 2010;341:c6895.
19. Amanzio M, Pollo A, Maggi G, Benedetti F. Response variability to analgesics: a role for non-specific activation of endogenous opioids. Pain. 2001;90:205–15.
20. Kirsch I, Deacon BJ, Huedo-Medina TB, et al. Initial severity and antidepressant benefits: a meta-analysis of data submitted to the Food and Drug Administration. PLoS Med. 2008;5:260–8.
21. Moncrieff J, Wessely S, Hardy R. Active placebos versus antidepressants for depression. Cochrane Database Syst Rev. 2004;1:CD003012.
22. Wartolowska K, Judge A, Hopewell S, et al. Use of placebo controls in the evaluation of surgery: systematic review. BMJ. 2014;348:g3253.
23. Moffet HH. Sham acupuncture may be as efficacious as true acupuncture: a systematic review of clinical trials. J Altern Complement Med. 2009;15:213–6.
24. Babel P, Bajcar EA, Adamczyk E, et al. Classical conditioning without verbal suggestions elicits placebo analgesia and nocebo hyperalgesia. PLoS One. 2017;12:e0181856.
25. Colloca L, Benedetti F. Placebo analgesia induced by social observational learning. Pain. 2009;144:28–34.
26. Kirchhof J, Petrakova L, Brinkhoff A, et al. Learned immunosuppressive placebo responses in renal patients. PNAS. 2018;115:4223–7.
27. Hall KT, Loscalzo J, Kaptchuk T. Pharmacogenomics and the placebo response. ACS Chem Neurosci. 2018;9:633–5.
28. Kashani A, Phillips CO, Foody JM, et al. Risk associated with statin therapy: a systematic overview of randomized clinical trials. Circulation. 2006;114:2788–97.
29. Gupta A, Thompson D, Whitehouse A, et al. Adverse events associated with unblended but not with blinded, statin therapy in Anglo-Scandinavian Cardiac Outcomes Trial-Lipid-Lowering Arm (ASCOT-LLA): a randomized double-blind placebo-controlled trial and its non-randomized non-blind extension phase. Lancet. 2017;389:2473–81.
30. Nielsen SF, Nordestgaard BG. Negative statin-related news stories decrease statin persistence and increase myocardial infarction and cardiovascular mortality: a nationwide prospective cohort study. Eur Heart J. 2016;37:908–16.
31. Matthews A, Herrett E, Gasparrini A, et al. Impact of statin related media coverage on use of statins: interrupted time series analysis with UK primary care data. BMJ. 2016;353:i3283.
32. Lionetti E, Pulvirenti A, Vallorani M, et al. Re-challenge studies in non-celiac gluten sensitivity: a systematic review and meta-analysis. Front Physiol. 2017;8:621.
33. Kirsch I. Response expectancy and the placebo effect. Int Rev Neurobiol. 2018;138:81–93.
34. Webster L, Albring A, Benson S, et al. Medicine related beliefs predict attribution of symptoms to a sham medicine: a prospective study. Br J Health Psychol. 2018;23:436–54.
35. Weissenfeld J, Stock S, Lungen M, Gerber A. The nocebo effect: a reason for patient's non-adherence to generic substitution. Pharmazie. 2010;65:451–6.
36. Witthöft M, Freitag I, Nussbaum C. On the origin of worries about modern health hazards: experimental evidence for a conjoint influence of media reports and personality traits. Psychol Health. 2018;33:361–80.
37. Roscoe JA, Morrow GR, Aapro MS, et al. Anticipatory nausea and vomiting. Support Care Cancer. 2011;19:1533–8.
38. Van den Bergh O, Winters W, Devriese S, Van Diest I. Learning subjective health complaints. Scand J Psychol. 2002;43:147–52.
39. Wientjes CJE, Grossman P. Over-reactivity of psyche or of the soma? Individual differences in psychosomatic symptoms, anxiety, heart rate and end -tidal partial carbon dioxide pressure. Psychosom Med. 1994;56(6):533–40.

40. Hornsveld HK, Garssen B, Dop MJ, et al. Double-blind placebo-control study of the hyperventilation provocation test and the validity of hyperventilation syndrome. Lancet. 1996;348:154–8.
41. Van den Bergh O, Brown R, Peterson S, Witthöft M. Idiopathic environmental intolerance: a comprehensive model. Clin Psychol Sci. 2017;5:551–67.
42. Genuis SJ. Chemical sensitivity: pathophysiology or pathopsychology? Clin Ther. 2013;35:572–7.
43. Dantoft TM, Andersson L, Nordin S, Skovbjerg S. Chemical intolerance. Curr Rheumatol Rev. 2015;11:167–84.
44. Steinemann A. Prevalence and effects of multiple chemical sensitivities in Australia. Prev Med Rep. 2018;10:191–4.
45. Bornschein S, Hausteiner C, Römmelt H, et al. Double-blind placebo-controlled provocation study in patients with subjective Multiple Chemical Sensitiviity (MCS) and matched control subjects. Clin Toxicol. 2008;46:443–9.
46. Nemery B, Fischler B, Boogaerts M, Lison D, Willems J. The Coca-Cola incident in Belgium, June 1999. Food Chem Toxicol. 2002;40:1657–67.
47. Nemery B, Fischler B, Boogaerts M, Lison D. Dioxins, Coca-Cola, and mass sociogenic illness in Belgium. Lancet. 1999;354:77.
48. Oftedal G, Wilén J, Sandström M, Mild KH. Symptoms experienced in connection with mobile phone use. Occup Med. 2000;50:237–45.
49. Roosli M, Moser M, Baldinini Y, Meier M, Braun-Fahrländer C. Symptoms of ill health ascribed to electromagnetic field exposure — a questionnaire survey. Int J Hyg Environ Health. 2004;207:141–50.
50. Rubin GJ, Das Munshi J, Wessely S. Electromagnetic hypersensitivity: a systematic review of provocation studies. Psychosom Med. 2005;67:224–32.
51. Rubin GJ, Hahn G, Everitt BS, Cleare AJ, Wessely S. Are some people sensitive to mobile phone signals? Within participants double-blind randomized provocation study. Br Med J. 2006;332:886–91.
52. Witthöft M, Rubin GJ. Are media warnings about the adverse health effects of modern life self-fulfilling? An experimental study on idiopathic environmental intolerance attributed to electromagnetic fields (IEI-EMF). J Psychosom Res. 2013;74:206–12.
53. Witthöft M, Rubin GJ. Are media warnings about the adverse health effects of modern life self-fulfilling? An experimental study on idiopathic environmental intolerance attributed to electromagnetic fields (IEI-EMF). J Psychosom Res. 2013;74:207.
54. Leventhall G. What is ultrasound? Prog Biophys Mol Biol. 2007;93:130–7.
55. Crichton F, Petrie KJ. Health complaints and wind turbines: the efficacy of explaining the nocebo response to reduce symptom reporting. Environ Res. 2015;140:449–55.
56. Knopper LD, Ollson CA. Health effects and wind turbines: a review of the literature. Environ Health. 2011;10:78.
57. Knopper LD, Ollson CA, McCallum LC, et al. Wind turbines and human health. Front Public Health. 2014;2:63.
58. Crichton F, Dodd G, Schmid G, Petrie KJ. Framing sound: using expectations to reduce environmental noise annoyance. Environ Res. 2015;142:609–14.
59. Karvala K, Sainio M, Palmquist E, et al. Building-related environmental intolerance and associated health in the general population. Int J Environ Res Public Health. 2018;15:2047–59.
60. Karvala K, Sainio M, Palmquist E, et al. Prevalence of various environmental intolerances in a Swedish and Finish general population. Environ Res. 2018;161:220–8.
61. Bogaerts K, Janssen T, De Peuter S, et al. Negative affective pictures can elicit physical symptoms in high habitual symptom reporters. Psychol Health. 2010;25:685–98.

Low Back Pain, Abdominal Pain and Headache

7

> *Pain is a cardinal manifestation of illness, and relief of pain is probably the most common demand made by the patient upon the physician. In spite of this importance of pain, it is astonishing how little we understand pain, but how confident we are of our knowledge of pain.*
>
> George Engel [1]

The notion that pain is not a primary sensation but rather an emotion, the opposite of pleasure, dominated the thinking of physicians and philosophers from the time of Hippocrates and Plato [2]. The prominent eighteenth century English physician Erasmus Darwin, grandfather of Charles Darwin, argued that pain was not a special sense since it could be produced by extreme stimulation of any of the senses, including the sensations of vision, hearing, touch, hot and cold. The eighteenth century English philosopher David Hartley felt that pain was pleasure carried beyond a due limit resulting from violent vibrations in the nerves and brain. Even after distinct pain nerves and brain pathways were identified in the latter part of the nineteenth century, physicians and researchers emphasized that the sensation of pain was not like other sensations. In the mid-twentieth century, the English neurologist William Gooddy pointed out that although impulse patterns in nerves and nerve centers in the brain provide the neurophysiological basis for pain and can influence the quality of pain, they do not determine whether or not an individual experiences pain [3]. There is a major psychological component to pain that is highly individual and influenced by past experience.

Pain is unique among body symptoms since it can be a warning signal of tissue damage. It is inherently frightening. When it is chronic, pain can become an illness in itself and have a major impact on a person's wellbeing. As many as 30–40% of the general population suffers from some type of chronic pain, and many of these

R. W. Baloh, *Medically Unexplained Symptoms*, https://doi.org/10.1007/978-3-030-59181-6_7

people take daily pain medications [4]. Chronic pain, defined as pain that lasts longer than 6 months, is the most common somatic symptom in American society. In 1980 more than 10 billion dollars were spent on disability payments to American patients with chronic pain problems. At the turn of the twenty-first century, an estimated 100 billion dollars per year was spent on treating chronic pain and 65 billion dollars per year was lost from missed work days due to chronic pain. Not only are patients with chronic pain a massive financial burden on the health care system and society but they personally are at high risk of being harmed from unnecessary tests, hospitalizations and surgeries.

Overview of Common Pain Syndromes

The three most common pain syndromes –low back pain, abdominal pain and headache – are ubiquitous in the general population. In most neurological practices, low back pain and headache are the most common reason for referral and in most of these people no organic structural cause can be identified. In a telephone survey published in 1989 of 10,200 randomly selected people between the ages of 12 and 29 in Washington County, Maryland, 77% of women and 57% of men reported having had a headache in the past month. In a report of 40 men with symptoms diagnosed as psychogenic in a Veterans Hospital in Minnesota in 1976, 58% had chronic pain other than headache and 32% had chronic headaches [5].

Low backache, abdominal pain and headache involve completely different parts of the body, yet they have features in common. Each can be caused by a potentially dangerous structural disorder, a benign musculoskeletal disorder, or a psychogenic disorder or some combination of the three. Considering the ominous implications of a structural disorder such as a herniated disc, appendicitis, or brain tumor, physicians tend to be very aggressive in evaluating patients with low back pain, abdominal pain and headache, particularly when they are new in onset. Yet most would agree that only a tiny fraction of these people have a serious cause. Should we obtain an MRI of the affected area in each person? Can society afford the costs of such tests? The answer to both questions is no, but often the decision with regard to testing depends more on the person's insurance than the clinical assessment. The presence of "red flags," worrisome associated symptoms or findings on examination should determine whether or not imaging is performed.

There is a balancing act between ruling out organic causes and identifying psychosocial factors. If one requires the absence of an organic cause, how much testing is required and when does testing stop and a decision made that an organic cause has been ruled out? On the other hand, the risk of focusing on psychological factors is that people with organic diseases may be labeled as psychogenic. One can see this dilemma with the evolving criteria for the diagnosis of psychogenic pain in sequential editions of the psychiatric diagnostic manual, the DSM (discussed in Chap. 4). In DSM III the diagnosis of psychogenic pain required that psychological factors were involved in causing the pain. There had to be a time relationship between the psychological factor and the onset or worsening of pain, and either the pain allowed the patient to avoid an undesirable activity or enabled the patient to obtain support that would otherwise not be available. These qualifiers suggested that the person might be using the pain for secondary gain, which is rarely the case. Even if secondary gain is involved, telling the person that their pain is not "real" will only aggravate the problem. The criteria were slightly modified in the DSM IV, but the basic structure remained the same. Critics of these diagnostic criteria pointed out that pain results from neurophysiological mechanisms gone awry and not from psychopathology. As our understanding of pain mechanisms have improved (discussed in Chap. 5), what previously seemed strange and unusual can now be explained. Furthermore, the psychological criteria are difficult to prove and their reliability has not been adequately tested in people with different pain disorders.

In response to these criticisms, the committee of psychiatrists working on DSM V decided to remove "psychogenic pain disorder" from the manual. It was replaced by a new broader category called "somatic symptom disorder," which essentially covers all psychosomatic symptoms, including pain [6]. Symptoms must be persistent and distressing and result in significant disruption of daily life. In addition, there must be disproportionate and persistent thoughts about the seriousness of the symptoms, a high level of anxiety about health, and excessive time and energy devoted to the symptoms or health concerns. Although these criteria emphasize important features of psychosomatic symptoms, they are of little use in managing patients with chronic pain. Critics immediately pointed out that with these broad criteria there is a good possibility of misdiagnosing a medical condition such as a herniated disc or rheumatoid arthritis as a psychogenic illness. Furthermore, just as with earlier criteria, adequate testing in sample populations was not performed before accepting the new criteria. Based on our current understanding of pain mechanisms, separation of organic and psychogenic causes of pain is inappropriate and unnecessary and may even be impossible, since pain by its very nature always has both organic and psychogenic elements.

Low Back Pain

Historical Perspective

For centuries, low back pain has been called lumbago, pain in the loins from the Latin word lumbus – loin. Lumbago was considered a type of rheumatism, from the Greek word rheuma, meaning a flux or flow. A watery discharge (evil humour) was thought to flow from the brain to the muscles and joints where it accumulated, causing inflammation and pain [7]. Lumbago was rheumatism involving the muscles of the low back caused by exposure to cold and damp. Well into the nineteenth century, physicians used a variety of treatments with the goal of removing the rheumatic humours from the affected muscles and joints. Although bloodletting, blistering and cupping were all used at times, liniments were most popular. Liniments were rubbed into the muscles of the back to create friction over the painful area. They were typically composed of an evaporating solvent such as alcohol or acetone, an analgesic such as camphor or capsaicin (an ingredient in chili peppers) and a counterirritant such as turpentine. The famous sixteenth century Swiss physician, Paracelsus (see Chap. 2), formulated the most widely known liniment, opodeldoc, a name derived from the variety of aromatic plants he used in the recipe [2]. Opodeldoc was made up of soap, alcohol, camphor and several herbal essences, including wormwood. It became the prototype for all future liniments. The humorous name "Old Opodeldoc" became synonymous with an old bumbling country doctor. Opodeldoc was popular in New England at the time of Edgar Allen Poe, who used the name opodeldoc for a character in his short story "The Literary Life of Thingum Bob, Esq." Remarkably, opodeldoc is still widely available in stores and on-line.

In the early nineteenth century, physicians first began focusing on the spine to explain low back pain. Brown's spinal irritation theory (discussed in Chap. 2) provided a mechanism for the spine and nerves to cause low back pain [7]. Irritation of nerves from the pelvic organs and areas on the skin of the back could trigger reflex pain in the back. Low back pain could be part of the generalized pain syndrome or a localized back pain syndrome. The story of Senator Charles Sumner's travails after his beating on the senate floor by the Southern congressman Preston Brooks in 1856 provides a nice glimpse of the impact of the spinal irritation theory on medical practice at the time [8]. After taking offense to an abolitionist speech by Sumner, Brooks attacked him with a cane, beating him unconscious. Sumner never fully recovered from the severe beating and he complained of severe pain when attempting to get up out of a chair and when walking. He also complained of chronic headaches and difficulty concentrating and focusing his attention. Several American physicians examined Sumner, but they could not identify a cause for his symptoms and felt that he was likely suffering from a psychogenic illness. More recently, some have speculated that he had the typical features of post-traumatic stress syndrome (PTSD) [9]. He was not able to return to his senate duties, and his doctors recommended rest and a sea voyage for "a complete separation from the cares and responsibilities that must beset him at home" [10]. He did show some improvement, at least in mood, with a trip to Europe, but his symptoms, particularly the severe pain, persisted and he could not return to the senate even after being reelected without campaigning. On a second trip to Europe in 1858, an American friend in Paris recommended that he see the world-renowned French-American neurologist Charles Edward Brown-Séquard, an expert on the spine (see Chap. 2). At the time, Paris was the mecca of the new rapidly advancing "scientific medicine." Brown-Séquard spent 3 hours examining Sumner in his hotel room and concluded that the beating had damaged several areas of Sumner's spine, and he recommended burning the skin over these areas with cotton soaked in a combustible substance. Sumner received six treatments from Brown-Séquard over 2 weeks. The pain was so intense that in the first session Sumner broke the chair he was gripping. Sumner suffered severe burns with the treatments, and it took months for him to recuperate. Even though many friends and physicians in America were appalled at what they considered a reckless treatment, Summer later wrote to his friend Henry Longfellow that without this cruel treatment he might have become an invalid, as Brown-Séquard warned [11].

The idea that low back pain might result from trauma to the spine evolved in the latter part of the nineteenth century. The industrial revolution and the rapid development of railway lines led to an increase in major traumatic injuries and the notion that low back pain could result from injury to the spine. Minor injuries accumulating over time, or even the constant jarring of the back associated with railway travel was also thought to lead to traumatic injury and development of low back pain. The condition called "Railway Spine" became a major public health concern, and governments responded with new compensation laws in the late 19th century that only compounded the problem [12]. Many people were given large lump sum payments for their disability. Proponents of railway spine suggested it was due to "concussion of the spine" or to decrease in blood flow to the spine [13]. Despite the lack of objective pathology in the spine, the idea that repetitive minor trauma could lead to severe permanent low back pain and disability was generally accepted by the both the lay public and medical-legal community at the turn of the twentieth century.

With the industrialization of Western societies in the early twentieth century, work-related injuries, chronic back pain and disability were increasing at an alarming rate. Industries attempted to hire workers who were physically fit, and working practices were modified to minimize back strain. With recruiting for the World War I, the military questioned whether development of back pain might be a fitness problem rather than a medical problem and developed special units to improve fitness for the many men who developed back pain during training exercises [14]. In World War II, chronic low back pain became the most common cause for hospitalization and withdrawal from active duty [15]. At this time, the concept of fibrositis, an inflammation of the fibrous tissue of the back, became popular to explain chronic low back pain. As we will see in the next chapter, fibrositis was also used to explain other chronic work-related injuries and more generalized body pain that evolved into the concept of fibromyalgia. After the World War II, a large medico-legal industry developed around the concept that chronic back pain due to repetitive trauma was a major cause of disability and that rest was the best treatment. This occurred even though the cause could not be identified in most cases and rest didn't seem to help.

In the mid-twentieth century, the notion that low back pain was commonly caused by degenerative changes in the spine became popular in both the lay and medical communities. In 1934 two surgeons at the Mass General Hospital in Boston, William Mixter and Joseph Barr, published a widely read paper on herniated intervertebral discs in the *New England Journal of Medicine* [16]. They convincingly showed that a ruptured disc could press on one of the lower spinal nerves as they exit the spinal canal, producing severe back pain radiating down the leg, so-called sciatica. Furthermore, they showed that surgical removal of the offending protruded disc cured the pain. Each intervertebral disc contains a gelatinous center surrounded by a fibrous band, which in turn is surrounded by a strong ligament [17]. With trauma and aging, degenerative arthritic changes occur in the gelatinous center and the surrounding fibrous disc. The gelatinous center slowly degrades from a resilient gel to a hardened substance. Disc protrusions (where the gelatinous center bulges through the fibrous disc but is held in check by the annular ligament) occur in more than 50% of normal people, particularly in the low back region. Pain can result from activation of nerve endings in the outer ligament, compression of a spinal nerve, or an inflammatory response triggered by chemicals released from the bulging disc. But what was the relevance of these degenerative changes in the vast majority of people with chronic low back pain without sciatica? As better imaging became possible first with computed tomography (CT) and then magnetic resonance imaging (MRI), it became apparent that everyone has degenerative changes in the spine and that the degree of the degenerative changes did not correlate with the severity of back pain [18]. Making matters even worse, the number of back surgeries for chronic low back pain was increasing exponentially, while the number of patients with chronic low back pain was also increasing at an alarming rate. Could back surgery be increasing the risk for developing chronic back pain [19]?

Current Approach to Chronic Low Back Pain

Nearly everyone experiences low back pain at some time, so not surprisingly, the impact on overall health care costs and costs to individuals is considerable [20]. A definitive diagnosis is possible in only about 20% of people with low back pain; most are labeled as non-specific low back pain (NSLBP) [21]. This is a real problem for the wide variety of medical disciplines that deal with these patients. How do you treat a condition when the cause is unknown? At the present time, most physicians recommend a conservative approach – keep active, continue with regular activities as much as possible, and use pain medications as little as possible [22]. There is general agreement that bed rest should be avoided as much as possible. With an acute injury, management should focus on getting the person mobile as quickly as possible. Manual therapies such as traction and manipulations are commonly used, but there are no definitive clinical trials proving that these treatments are more effective than conservative management for NSLBP. Several clinical trials have concluded that traction is of no benefit, even in patients with objective evidence of nerve root impingement. Another dilemma with NSLBP is whether or not to image the low back. Routine x-rays are rarely useful. CT and MRI are more useful, but the increased sensitivity can be a problem since ubiquitous "disc disease" often has nothing to do with the patient's symptoms [23]. Surgery on the back, particularly when the indication for surgery is not absolutely clear, is a major risk factor for developing chronic low back pain.

Since chronic low back pain is often resistant to treatment, patients become frustrated with traditional medical care and seek alternative treatments. Most patients can accept the uncertainty of diagnosis, but it is critical that they perceive that they are being taken seriously [24]. NSLBP has many risk factors. A kind of priming of the pump occurs such that people who have had pain experiences in the past are more susceptible to developing chronic pain. As described in Chap. 5, central sensitization is a process whereby an episode of pain triggers increased sensitivity to pain through a variety of complex changes in the chemistry and connectivity of brain pathways. Psychosocial factors play a critical role in determining whether or not one develops chronic low back pain. Social networks, level of routine activity and expectations all affect the risk for developing chronic back pain. Numerous studies have found a high rate of comorbidity of depression, somatization, anxiety and stress in patients with chronic low back pain [25]. Finally, variations in genes that code for key proteins within the brain pain pathways have been shown to increase pain sensitivity in humans and in several animal models [26].

Physical Activity and Expectation

There is convincing evidence that regular physical activity, whether a structured exercise program or exercise associated with leisure activities, decreases the risk for developing chronic low back pain [27]. On the other hand, "catastrophizing," always expecting the worst, increases the disability associated with chronic back pain (the nocebo effect discussed in Chap. 6). If one anticipates a catastrophic consequence of an activity such as exercise, one will avoid the activity. People need constant reassurance that activities such as exercise are not causing their chronic low back pain. Just the opposite, inactivity is a clear risk factor for developing chronic low back pain [28]. Since pain normally signals impending danger or harm, it is not surprising that patients with pain might avoid activities such as exercise that can induce or exacerbate pain. While this may be an appropriate reaction to acute pain, fear-avoidance behavior can lead to increased disability with chronic low back pain. Muscles become weak, joints become stiff and bones become thinner. Regular exercise is absolutely necessary for successful living with chronic low back pain (see Chap. 10). Although any exercise is better than none, a combination strengthening and stretching of the back along with aerobic exercise three times per week is recommended.

Depression and Fear Avoidance

Of the various psychogenic illnesses, depression has received the most study and has the clearest relationship with chronic low back pain [29, 30]. There is a bidirectional relationship between low back pain and depression – low back pain causes depression and depressed subjects are more likely to develop chronic low back pain. It isn't hard to imagine why chronic low back pain causes depression for anyone who has experienced chronic back pain. It is difficult to enjoy normally pleasurable activities when experiencing constant back pain. One becomes preoccupied with the pain. Fear of pain may be a better predictor of chronic disability than the degree of pain itself [31]. Fear of the long-term consequences of surgery predicts those who develop chronic postoperative pain. Anxiety- and neuroticism-prone subjects are more likely to develop the vicious cycle of fear and pain. Understanding how this vicious cycle occurs can help people break the cycle of chronic low back pain.

Abdominal Pain

Abdominal pain, like low back pain, is extremely common in the general population. When acute, a range of potentially dangerous diseases such as appendicitis, peptic ulcers, inflammatory bowel disease and cancer must be considered. Less dangerous but equally painful causes include muscle and tendon strains and tears. With chronic abdominal pain, psychogenic factors are more important [32]; some of these people have just pain, while others have a combination of abdominal pain and abnormalities in bowel motility – the irritable bowel syndrome (IBS). Many people with chronic abdominal pain, particularly those with IBS, eagerly seek surgery, so it is important to consider structural pathology and identify psychogenic factors early to prevent needless surgery. Just as with low back pain, surgery itself is a risk factor for developing and maintaining chronic abdominal pain.

Autonomic Nervous System and the Gut

The body's internal organs, including the gut, are controlled by a separate nervous system, the autonomic nervous system, whose nerve cell bodies are located in a series of ganglia located along the vertebral column. The idea of two different nervous systems, one in charge of voluntary behavior and the other in charge of vegetative processes dates back to the late eighteenth century. In his famous book *Recherches physiologiques sur la vie and la mort* (Physiological researches upon life and death) the French anatomist and physiologist Marie François Xavier Bichat noted that vegetative functions such as circulation, intestinal absorption and glandular secretion often continue after brain death [33]. He concluded that there were two lives, the animal life and the vegetative life. In some patients with severe brain injuries, animal life (conscious and voluntary activities) stopped, while vegetative life (activity in the deep internal organs) continued. Anatomical studies showed that the deep internal organs received almost no cerebral nerves but many nerves from the ganglionic nervous system (the series of small independent "brains" in the chest cavity along the vertebral column –called the sympathetic nervous system). The term "sympathetic" can be traced to the ancient concept of nervous sympathy between the deep internal body organs. The autonomic nervous system would much later be divided into sympathetic and parasympathetic components based on different functions and different neurotransmitters.

Early surgeons concluded that there must be a sympathetic sensibility since patients reported severe pain if the sympathetic ganglia were inadvertently touched or damaged during surgery [34]. An example of sympathetic mediated pain is the intense chest pain (angina) that occurs with a heart attack. Removing the sympathetic ganglia supplying the heart relieves the pain. Activation of the sympathetic nervous system causes pain but, even more important, activation of the sympathetic system modulates pain and triggers secondary changes in the blood circulation in the area of the pain. Pain fibers coming from the internal organs run in peripheral nerves and special sympathetic nerves called splanchnic nerves to the sympathetic ganglia and then back to the spinal nerves to enter the spinal cord so injury to any of these structures can activate visceral pain fibers [35]. Pain activation of the sympathetic system can lead to a variety of secondary tissue changes, including changes in temperature, swelling, changes in skin texture and color and local sweating. The unconscious mind can control what the conscious mind cannot – the internal organs such as the heart and bowels. Pain signals reaching the limbic system can trigger the hypothalamic pituitary adrenal axis, providing a generalized activation of the sympathetic system along with fear and anxiety. This mechanism explains panic reactions with racing of the heart, chest pressure, increased motility of the gut, and a smothering sensation. Many of these secondary symptoms are frightening and confusing and can lead to a vicious cycle of fear and anxiety.

The complex interrelationship between the mind and the bowels has baffled physicians for several hundred years. In 1816, the German physician, G. L. Hohnstock described a bowel-obsessed patient with chronic symptoms of constipation, diarrhea and abdominal pain typical of modern-day irritable bowel syndrome (IBS). Hohnstock wrote, "he directs his attention very specifically to his B.M.'s because what agony and anxiety constipation cause him. Whenever the subject comes around to constipation socially, he perceives again these hypochondriacal complaints. He is happy to spend long sessions upon the toilet. To extend his stay he lays in a supply of books. Also, he takes purgatives to combat constipation, and any doctor can insinuate himself with [the patient] who is willing to prescribe them.... The hypochondriac now believes that life is impossible without laxatives, and if none are available, he gives himself an enema. He also pays quite exact notice to his stool and its composition, keeps a diary of it in which he records daily with great exactness the quantity and quality of the excrement" [36]. Although Dr. Hohnstock's patient may have been a hypochondriac with psychogenic symptoms, he also had a clear gut motility disorder.

Irritable Bowel Syndrome (IBS)

IBS nicely illustrates the complex relationship between organic and psychic factors in the production of chronic pain. IBS is characterized by a combination of chronic abdominal pain and alterations in gut motility [37]. The abnormal motility can be diarrhea-predominant (IBS-D), constipation dominant (IBS-C) or alternating between diarrhea and constipation (IBS-A). Genetic, environmental and psychogenic factors all play a role in the cause of IBS. Increased incidence of IBS in twins and multigenerational families confirms a genetic substrate for IBS. The syndrome is polygenetic, with some gene variations increasing the risk of developing IBS while others decreasing the risk. Several other neurological disorders with a major psychogenic component occur with greater frequency in patients with IBS than in the general population (comorbidities); up to 50% of patients with IBS have migraine, chronic fatigue syndrome, fibromyalgia and depression [38]. IBS is triggered by a gastrointestinal infection in a small percentage of cases. Release of inflammatory cytokines during the acute infection may damage the gut epithelial barrier, increasing permeability, a consistent feature of IBS. Patients with IBS have high levels of anxiety, suggesting possible abnormalities in the stress response system – the hypothalamic-pituitary-adrenal axis and the sympathetic nervous system (see Chap. 5). Studies have found that psychogenic illness (particularly anxiety and depression) precedes the onset of IBS in as many as two-thirds of patients [39].

Peptic Ulcer Disease

Few diseases better illustrate the complex interrelationship between organic and psychogenic mechanisms for the production of symptoms than peptic ulcer disease. The excruciating upper abdominal pain associated with peptic ulcers has been recognized for centuries, but it wasn't until the beginning of the twentieth century that the correlation between acid secretion in the stomach and the formation of peptic ulcers was recognized [40]. By the end of the nineteenth century, there was conclusive evidence that the stomach secreted hydrochloric acid along with digestive enzymes and that acid secretion increased with stress and emotional upset. U.S. Army surgeon William Beaumont performed one of the earliest studies of gastric secretions in a patient with a gastric fistula who he followed for almost a decade beginning in 1822. Beaumont was stationed at Fort Mackinac on Mackinac Island, Michigan, where he treated French-Canadian trapper Alexis St. Martin after he had been shot point-blank in the abdomen. St. Martin slowly recovered, but he was left with an inch and a half-scarred opening between the skin over the abdomen and his stomach. Through the fistula, for years Beaumont monitored gastric secretions in a variety of circumstances and published the results in a book entitled Experiments and Observations on the Gastric Juice and the Physiology of Digestion in 1833 [41].

German surgeon Karl Schwartz provided the definitive linkage between peptic ulcers and acid secretion when he published a series of 14 patients operated upon to remove peptic ulcers in 1910 [42]. He noted that ulcers only occurred in the esophagus, stomach, and upper intestines, the only areas where acid was present. He coined the famous phrase "Ohne sauerenMagensaft kein peptisches Geschwür," or in English, "no acid no ulcer." From that time, the management of peptic ulcers focused on controlling gastric hydrochloric acid production [43]. Surgeons performed a wide variety of procedures to decrease acid production, including cutting the vagus nerve, and pharmacists developed medications to neutralize stomach acid. In America, people carried Tums with them to treat their daily indigestion and heartburn and hopefully prevent the development of peptic ulcers. A pharmacist in St. Louis, Missouri, James Howe, invented Tums in his basement for his wife's chronic indigestion, and he teamed up with his uncle, who was also a pharmacist, to form the Lewis-Howe Company to produce Tums in 1930. Tums is an antacid, calcium carbonate ($CaCO_3$), in a chewable tablet. It is still produced in the original factory in Missouri recently renovated by GlaxoSmithKline. Advertising with the slogan "Tums for the tummy" was a major factor in the widespread popularity of Tums. There was a general acceptance in the medical community and among the lay public that stress increased hydrochloric acid production, so in addition to antacids, patients with peptic ulcers were often treated with a restful period away from work and stressful activities. I still have vivid memories of an uncle who suffered from recurrent peptic ulcers in the mid-twentieth century. He had been in World War II and suffered severe frostbite in the Battle of the Bulge, so when he returned home and began experiencing typical ulcer pain, everyone, including his family doctor, attributed the ulcers to the stress from his war experiences. With each ulcer exacerbation, he was confined to bed for several days to rest while taking Tums and milk every few hours to soothe his pain. He was a strong man, and the stigma that an emotional weakness was somehow contributing to his condition bothered him as much as his symptoms.

By the mid-twentieth century, there was a general consensus: peptic ulcers were caused by excessive stomach acid production and stress and emotional upset were behind the excessive acid production. But this would all dramatically change with the discovery by two Australian physicians, Robin Warren, a pathologist and Barry Marshall, a gastroenterologist, that a bacterium, *Helicobactor pylori*, could cause peptic ulcers. Warren had noticed bacteria associated with an intense immune response in gastric biopsy specimens in the early 1970s, but it wasn't until he published his findings in 1983 that Marshall suggested that the bacterium might be the cause of peptic ulcers [44, 45]. To prove that the bacteria caused disease, Marshall inoculated himself with the stomach contents of a 66-year-old patient with peptic ulcer disease [46]. Marshall developed gastrointestinal symptoms, and endoscopic biopsy of his stomach showed *H. pylori* and evidence of gastritis. Understandably, there was initially great skepticism regarding Marshall's findings, but over the subsequent years he and others convinced the medical community that *H. pylori* could cause peptic ulcers and that antibiotics could cure patients with peptic ulcers. Research studies on *H. pylori* showed that it had a unique ability to live in the acid-rich stomach and produce molecules that allowed it to adhere to the stomach lining and toxins that induced a strong immune response, damaging the stomach and intestinal lining [47].

Around the same time, it became apparent that there was another common risk factor for the development of peptic ulcers, nonsteroidal anti-inflammatory drugs (NSAIDs). It had long been known that aspirin (acetylsalicylic acid), particularly in high doses, could irritate the stomach and intestines and was a common cause of gastrointestinal bleeding, initially attributed to aspirin's acidic properties. This led to the development of newer NSAIDs such as ibuprofen (Advil) and naproxen (Aleve) that were considered less irritating to the gastrointestinal lining. But with widespread use of these newer NSAIDs, it became apparent that they could also damage the gastrointestinal lining and predispose to development of peptic ulcers [48]. By systemic inhibition of prostaglandins, all NSAIDs impair mucous production, bicarbonate secretion and the ability of the lining to repair itself after injury. Furthermore, there likely is a synergistic interaction between *H. pylori* and NSAIDs in the production of peptic ulcers since both can damage the gastrointestinal lining [49]. By the turn of the twenty-first century, there was a consensus that acid played only a secondary role in producing peptic ulcers. The gastrointestinal lining must first be injured by either NSAIDs or *H. pylori*. The role of stress was largely relegated to a minor contributing factor. But then the pendulum began to swing back in the opposite direction after large epidemiological studies conducted in Scandinavia showed that stress plays an important role in the production of peptic ulcers regardless of *H. pylori* infection or NSAID use [50]. In a study of 223,093 Swedish men, decreased ability to handle stress was associated with a significantly increased risk of developing peptic ulcers, and in a study of 17,525 residents in northern Denmark followed for 33 months, those with the highest perceived daily stress level were more than twice as likely to receive treatment for *H. pylori* or be diagnosed with peptic ulcers than those with the lowest perceived daily stress level [51, 52]. Stress could also influence the healing and recurrence rate of peptic ulcers [53]. Complicating matters even further, recent studies show that genetic risk factors are important both for developing *H. pylori* infection and for developing peptic ulcers independent of *H. pylori* infection [54]. So similar to most other psychosomatic illnesses, peptic ulcers have a complicated combination of risk factors [55], with the main risk factors being *H. pylori* infection, NSAID use, susceptibility genes and psychological stress. Lesser risk factors include smoking, excessive alcohol use, acid production, and obesity, all of which individually are dependent on the levels of daily stress.

Primary Headache Disorders

As with back pain, just about everyone has experienced a headache at some time in his or her life; in some people, headaches are chronic and disabling. There are two common primary headache disorders: tension-type headaches and migraine headaches. Both of these headache disorders can become chronic and occur daily, particularly when pain medications are used daily, producing so-called medication overuse headache. Primary headache disorder means that the headaches are a primary illness and not due to some other neurological disorder. Although there are several differences between these two types of headaches, the main difference is pain severity; migraine headaches are typically more severe and restrict activities more than tension-type headaches. Both types of headache can be disabling and lead to lost work days. Migraine headaches are often throbbing and one-sided and are associated with nausea and/or light and sound sensitivity, whereas tension-type headaches are on both sides, described as pressing or tightness and are not associated with nausea and usually do not have light or sound sensitivity. Both types of headaches can last from hours to days, although tension-type headaches tend to be shorter in duration. Finally, both types of headaches can occur in the same person and both are triggered by a variety of psychogenic factors [56].

Tension-type headaches are the most common type of headache, with a lifetime prevalence of about 70% in men and 90% in women, so just about everyone has had one at some time. By contrast, the lifetime prevalence of migraine headaches is about 5% in men and 15% in women. Medication-overuse headache is caused by mistreatment of tension-type or migraine headaches; it does not occur separately. About 75% of cases of medication overuse headache occur in people with migraine while about 25% occur in people with tension-type headaches. Because of the high prevalence of tension-type headaches, the overall cost and disability in society is about the same for tension-type headaches and migraine headaches, even though migraine headaches are typically much more severe. In one population study, patients with tension-type headaches reported an average of 9 lost work days and 5 days in which they experienced decreased efficiency every year. In a European study on the global burden of disease, migraine was the number-one cause of disability in the age group 15–49, a time frame many would consider the most productive years in a person's life [57]. The most conspicuous precipitating factor for both tension-type and migraine headaches is stress. Other common triggers are alcohol, caffeine withdrawal, weather (barometric) changes and menstruation. Sleep disturbances are common with both types of headaches. Improvement of the headache during pregnancy is more frequent with migraine than with tension-type headaches.

Depression is tightly interrelated with both migraine and tension-type headaches. As with low back pain, there is a bidirectional relationship between migraine and depression; people with depression are at increased risk of developing migraine headaches, and people with migraine headaches are at increased risk of developing depression. This observation suggests that there is a shared mechanism for these common disorders. The relationship of depression and tension-type headaches is more complex, but clearly there is an increased incidence of depression in patients with chronic tension-type headaches (15 or more days of headaches a month). Tension-type headache sufferers have central sensitization to pain in cranial tissues, and depression further increases the central sensitization to pain (see Chap. 5) [58].

Migraine as a Model for Psychophysiological Illnesses

The British-born American neurologist and writer Oliver Sachs nicely summarized the complexity of migraine in his 1970 book *Migraine: Evolution of a Common Disorder.* "A migraine [headache] expresses both physiological and emotional needs: it is the prototype of a psychophysiological reaction. Thus, the convergence of thinking which its understanding demands must be based simultaneously both on neurology and psychiatry…" [59]. Understanding the mechanism of migraine provides a window into understanding all psychosomatic illnesses, which are in fact psychophysiological illnesses, meaning the symptoms are caused by the mind altering the physiology of the brain.

Historical Perspective

Migraine headaches have been recognized for thousands of years and have been given many different names: heterocrania, hemicrania, bilious headache, sick headache, blind headache, megrim and migraine. The celebrated Greek physician Aretaeus provided the best early description of migraine, which he called heterocrania, "an illness by no means mild…It occasions unseemly and dreadful symptoms…nausea; vomiting of bilious matters; collapse of the patient…there is much torpor, heaviness of the head, anxiety; and life becomes a burden. For they flee the light; the darkness soothes their disease; nor can they bear readily to look upon or hear anything pleasant… The patients are weary of life and wish to die" [60]. Based on the humoral theory of disease popular at the time, Aretaeus and his fellow Greek physicians thought that migraine headaches resulted from excessive yellow or black bile producing a bilious humour that moved through the body causing the vomiting and stomach upset associated with a sick headache. Constipation could cause the stomach and bowels to become laden with bilious humors, so emetics and laxatives were commonly used as treatment. "Liver pills" were used to decrease the bilious humors at their source and bloodletting could diminish their concentration in the blood. Interestingly, even in these early times physicians were aware of a potential role for diet in triggering migraine headaches and recommended avoiding fatty foods, which were thought to draw bilious humors to the stomach [61].

The seventeenth century physician Thomas Willis (see Chap. 2) published the first major treatise on headache in two chapters in his famous book *De Anima Brutorom.* In the book, Willis described migraine headaches suffered by a "Nobel Lady" that he had been following for years, "The sickness being limited to no one place on the head, troubled her sometimes on one side, sometimes on the other, and often thorow the whole compass of the Head. During the fit (which rarely ended under a day and a night's space, and often held for two, three, or four days) she was impatient of light, speaking, noise, or any motion, sitting upright in her Bed, the Chamber made dark, she would talk to nobody, nor take any sleep, or sustenance. At length about the declination of the fit, she was wont to lye down with an heavy and disturbed sleep, from which awakening she found herself better…" [62]. Willis captured the major features of migraine headaches, including sensitivity to any kind of movement, whether of the self or surround, and the importance of sleep in breaking the headache cycle.

Willis was the first to hint at a vascular theory for migraine with vasoconstriction followed by vasodilatation, a theory that became popular in the 19th and early 20th centuries. He recognized the importance of innate (hereditary) constitutional factors and suggested that irritation of an internal organ such as the uterus, spleen and stomach could set off a migraine headache, a type of organ "sympathy." The autonomic nervous system was unknown at the time, but Willis suggested some type of nervous interaction between these different organs. For treatment of migraine headaches, Willis recommended feverfew and the newly introduced coffee, treatments still commonly used for migraine. He emphasized that the headaches often occurred in distinct patterns at certain times of the day, in different seasons and with changes in weather.

Migraine Auras

Migraine auras were recognized for many centuries, but it wasn't until the nineteenth century that the relationship between aura and migraine was appreciated. Migraine auras can take on several forms, including visual distortions and hallucinations, sensory loss, muscle weakness, difficulty speaking and cognitive impairment. They can precede a migraine headache or occur independent of headache. Many famous physicians, scientists, writers and artists through the years have had migraine visual auras and many wrote about and drew the auras, particularly when they occurred in isolation. The nineteenth century English physician Hubert Airy provided detailed descriptions of the scintillating scotoma that he experienced prior to his migraine headaches. "A bright stellate object, a small angled sphere, suddenly appears in one side of the combined field…it rapidly enlarges, first as a circular zigzag, but on the inner side, towards the medial line, the regular outline becomes faint, and, as the increase in size goes on, the outline here becomes broken…the lines which constitute the outline meet at right angles or larger angles…" [63]. The scotoma was a shadowy area of blindness that trailed behind the scintillating zigzag crescent that Airy described as having gorgeous chromatic edgings. Unfortunately for Airy, this spectacular personal show of fireworks meant that a terrible headache would soon follow.

Some of the "visions" reported by early religious figures almost certainly represented migraine visual aura without headache. One of the best documented cases of a migraine visual aura being interpreted as a religious experience was Hildegard of Bingen, a twelfth century nun and mystic. She had "visions" throughout her life that she documented with drawings and detailed descriptions later in life. She observed points of light that shimmered and moved in waves that she interpreted as stars or flaming eyes. "The visions which I saw I beheld neither in sleep, nor in dreams, nor in madness, nor with my carnal eyes, nor with the ears of the flesh, nor in hidden places; but wakeful, alert, and with the eyes of the spirit …Sometimes I behold within this light another light which I name 'the Living Light itself'…And when I look upon it every sadness and pain vanishes from my memory, so that I am again as a simple maid and not as an old woman" [64].

The term "Alice in Wonderland syndrome" was coined in 1955 by the British psychiatrist John Todd to describe a type of visual hallucination called metamorphopsia that can occur with a migraine aura but can also be seen with other brain disorders [65]. As part of a migraine aura, patients experience bizarre distortions of their physical world. The name was derived from Lewis Carroll's children's book *Alice's Adventures in Wonderland* in which Alice experienced a variety of physical distortions such as feeling that her body and objects around her were growing larger and smaller. There has been a great deal of interest as to whether Carroll received his inspiration to write *Alice Adventures in Wonderland* and its sequel *Through the Looking Glass* based on his own experience with migraine aura, which he had had throughout his life, mostly without headaches and beginning before he had written the books [66]. He had consulted with ophthalmologists for his strange visual experiences, but no diagnosis was made until he read an article on migraine aura by Peter Latham, published in the British Medical Journal in 1872 (a year after *Through the Looking Glass* was published).

Early Ideas on the Cause of Migraine

In the early 1870s, two physicians at Cambridge University in London, Edward Liveing and Peter Latham, wrote separate monographs on migraine, each proposing a different mechanism for migraine symptoms, the neuronal theory and the vascular theory [67]. These two broad theories have dominated thinking on migraine since that time, and current ideas on migraine mechanisms contain features of both theories. In *On Megrim, Sick-Headaches and Some Allied Disorders,* Liveing provided detailed descriptions of 60 patients with migraine from his own practice and other sources, the first comprehensive look at the breadth of the "migraine experience." He emphasized the diversity of symptoms with migraine, including a variety of headache and aura patterns. He was the first to describe episodic vertigo with migraine. Oliver Sachs noted that *On Megrim* was a "treasure of clinical observations; such a mingling, at once, of intellectual passion and human feeling; so riveting, so genial, so easily and naturally written...crucial for the generation of my own thoughts" [68]. At the time of Liveing, the distinction between medical writing and popular writing was not as great as in modern times. Indeed, it was Sach's unique ability to cross the boundary between medical and popular writing that propelled his highly successful career as a popular medical writer, undoubtedly the most widely read neurologist of all times.

With inductive reasoning commonly used by physicians of his time, Liveing concluded that migraine resulted from a "nerve-storm" analogous to other similar paroxysmal disorders such as epilepsy [69]. In the case of a migraine visual aura, Liveing suggested that the nerve-storm began in the visual thalamus (a key visual relay station deep in the brain) and then moved from above downwards, or from before backwards. He proposed a spread of nervous excitation with migraine similar to the spread of epileptic activity along the motor cortex with focal motor seizures that his contemporary, Hughlings Jackson, would propose a few years later. Had Liveing chosen the visual cortex rather than the visual thalamus for the origin of the "nerve-storm," his theory might have had more lasting impact but as presented it was largely forgotten by future researchers on the mechanism of migraine. In Liveing's defense, little was known about cerebral cortical localization at the time.

While Liveing developed his theory of migraine purely based on clinical observations, Peter Latham developed his theory based on a combination of clinical observations and laboratory work on the sympathetic nervous system of rabbits that he conducted at Downing College at Cambridge [70]. Latham cut the nerves from the sympathetic ganglia supplying the rabbit's neck and noted that electrical stimulation of the cut nerves caused the blood vessels to constrict and then dilate. He hypothesized that with migraine the brain lost its normal regulating power over the sympathetic ganglia and "instead of tranquil, even, harmonious action in the various organs, as in perfect health, we have convulsive, excited and painful movements" [71]. Latham speculated that the migraine aura was caused by excitement of the sympathetic nerves causing vascular constriction and that the headache was caused by the reactive vascular dilatation. Although others, including Thomas Willis, had considered a possible vascular origin for migraine, Latham provided the most detailed theory of the time. Liveing was an early critic of Latham's vascular theory, pointing out that if vascular constriction and the associated decreased blood flow to the brain was a necessary forerunner of the subsequent vascular dilatation and headache, why did so many attacks simply consist of headache and why did the aura often continue into the headache phase.

The idea that migraine might have a vascular origin remained dormant for more than a half century when in the 1930s American neurologist Harold Wolff conducted seminal experiments in patients with migraine at the Cornell Medical Center in New York and reinvented the vascular theory of migraine. After completing medical school at Harvard and an internship in New York, Wolff returned to Harvard from 1926 to 1928 to work as a research fellow with Stanley Cobb, the pioneer biological psychiatrist who believed that there was no distinction between functional and organic disease [72]. After completing fellowship training in Europe with Nobel laureates Otto Loewi in Austria and Ivan Pavlov in Russia and in Baltimore at Johns Hopkins Hospital with psychiatrist Adolf Meyer, Wolff took the post of chief neurologist at the newly established Cornell Medical Center with the goal of understanding the borderland between functional and organic diseases. He chose to study migraine because it seemed to be the ideal disease to investigate the interaction between the psyche and biology in producing nervous disorders. At Cornell, Wolff developed methods to measure intracranial and extracranial blood flow changes during a migraine attack and noted that a migraine aura could be temporarily aborted with a drug that caused dilatation of blood vessels increasing blood flow to the brain. He gave a medical student who was experiencing a typical migraine scintillating scotoma a whiff of amyl nitrate, a vasodilating drug used to treat cardiac angina, and the scotoma transiently disappeared only to return as the drug wore off. On the other hand, he could abort the headache phase of migraine by giving a patient ergotamine tartrate, a drug known to cause constriction of blood vessels and decrease blood flow. Based on these observations, Wolff concluded that migraine aura resulted from vasoconstriction of intracranial blood vessels causing decreased blood flow to areas of the brain such as the visual cortex, and migraine headaches were caused by vasodilation of the extracranial blood vessels activating pain fibers in the walls of the blood vessels. Wolff's vascular theory improved upon Latham's theory and provided a potential new treatment for migraine headaches, ergotamine. Interestingly, in his now classic textbook *Headache and Other Head Pain,* first published in 1948, Wolff outlined his vascular theory in detail but did not mention Latham or any prior vascular theories of migraine [73].

Wolff, who had migraine himself, thought that people who were highly successful, ambitious, and perfectionist, a so-called migraine personality, were more prone to develop migraine than other people. Although this theory has largely been debunked, it can probably be traced to his seeing successful, affluent patients from the Upper East Side of Manhattan and his own perfectionist tendencies. Wolff felt that highly successful people placed unrealistic expectations upon themselves, producing tension that caused vasoconstriction of intracranial arteries and fatigue that caused vasodilatation of extracranial arteries. Analogous to Beard's theory on the cause of neurasthenia, Wolff proposed that migraine was the cranial vascular consequence of a stressful way of life. Like many before him, Wolff identified large families with migraine and emphasized the importance of hereditary factors in migraine susceptibility. Helen Goodell, Wolff's research assistant at Cornell, nicely summarized Wolff's overview of migraine: "Migraine headaches commonly occur when hereditarily susceptible persons attempt to control feelings of anxiety and resentment by means of organized and intense activity" [74].

Mechanism of the Migraine Aura

At about the same time Wolff was developing his vascular theory of migraine, a new neuronal theory of migraine was taking shape based on a combination of clinical and laboratory observations. In 1941, Karl Lashley, a well-known psychologist on the faculty at Harvard University, published an article in *Archives of Neurology and Psychiatry* in which he reported a series of sketches of his own migraine visual aura over time and concluded that "a wave of intense excitation is propagated at a rate of 3 mm per minute across the visual cortex. This wave is followed by complete inhibition of activity, with recovery progressing at the same rate" [75]. Lashley had studied the cellular architecture of the cerebral cortex in a variety of animals, including primates, and he had a particular interest in the visual cortex (occipital cortex) and the study of color vision. Over several years, Lashley mapped a large number of his migraine aura that occurred isolated from headache or any other symptoms. He wrote, "The scotoma usually occurs first as a small blind or scintillating spot, subtending less than 1 degree, in or immediately adjacent to the foveal field [central vision]. This spot rapidly increases in size and drifts away from the fovea toward the temporal field of one side. Usually both quadrants of one side only are involved, the right and left being affected with about equal frequency" [76]. To map the developing scotoma in his visual field, Lashley placed a dot on a white piece of paper and while focusing on the dot he moved a pencil toward the developing scintillating scotoma from different directions and marked the position on the paper where the pencil disappeared. He kept repeating the process at fixed time intervals to map the changing size of the scotoma. Lashley estimated the 3 mm rate of spread across the visual cortex assuming that the "disturbance" began near the occipital pole and moved toward the temporal margin (a distance of about 67 mm) in about 20 min (the typical duration of the aura). He speculated that scintillations on the rim of the scotoma represented a wave of intense excitation of the visual cortex followed by a wave of total inhibition, the blind area.

At the time of Lashley's report, a young Brazilian physiologist, Aristides Leão, was working on his doctorate at Harvard Medical School, which he received in 1943. In the following year, based on his doctoral thesis, Leão published an article in the *Journal of Neurophysiology* describing a curious phenomenon that he called, cortical spreading depression [77]. The article would become one of the most widely quoted articles in the history of neuroscience and provide a conceptual basis for understanding the mechanism of migraine. Leão's basic observation was that he could trigger a slowly propagating wave of depression of electrical activity in the cerebral cortex of a rabbit, pigeon or cat with a pinpoint electrical or mechanical stimulus and that the wave of depression moved across the cortex at a rate of between 2 and 5 mm/min. In a second article in the same journal he reported that the wave of depression was associated with dilatation and constriction of the tiny arteries overlying the cortical area with the depressed electrical activity [78]. This observation suggested a close interrelationship between neuronal activity and cerebral blood flow (now considered the neurovascular unit) and a potential link between the neural and vascular theories of migraine. Leão returned to Rio de Janeiro in 1947 where he continued to study and report on cortical spreading depression and where he developed a Laboratory of Biophysics that would become one of the most famous biophysical institutes in the world.

Genetic Susceptibility to Migraine

Another piece of the puzzle regarding the mechanism of migraine came with recent genetic studies in families with migraine. Familial occurrence of migraine has been well documented for centuries, but in most cases the pattern of transmission within families is complex, suggesting the likelihood of multiple different genes interacting to determine susceptibility [79]. However, rare families have been identified in which migraine is transmitted from generation to generation consistent with a single dominant gene causing the disorder. These families have a type of migraine called hemiplegic migraine in which affected members have auras consisting of hemiplegia, one-sided weakness or paralysis. Within these families, some members just have typical migraine visual aura and headache, but most have hemiplegic episodes at some time. So far mutations in three different genes have been identified that cause hemiplegic migraine, and all three genes code for channels that control the movement of ions such as sodium, potassium and calcium in and out of nerve cells leading to increased neuronal excitability. The most widely studied of these genes, codes for a calcium channel that is key for excitatory neurotransmission in the brain. This calcium ion channel is located in the nerve terminal of excitatory synapses throughout the brain and is key for release of the main excitatory neurotransmitter, glutamate (see Chap. 5). When the nerve impulse reaches the synapse, the change in voltage opens the calcium channel, allowing calcium to enter the nerve terminal and set off the cascade of events that leads to the release of tiny packets of glutamate. Glutamate then crosses the synapse and excites the next nerve cell in the chain of excitation. In animal models, mutations in the gene like those that occur in patients with hemiplegic migraine decrease the threshold for triggering cortical spreading depression. In other words, the spreading depression is triggered much more easily than in animals without the mutation. Detailed recording of the spreading depression in these animals show a leading edge of excitation followed by a wide area of depolarization of nerve cells and complete absence of electrical activity [80]. Furthermore, functional MRI studies measuring cerebral blood flow in patients experiencing a migraine aura fit nicely with the spreading depression theory.

Our current understanding of migraine involves a complex interaction of genetic, environmental and psychological factors that can set off a wave of excitation followed by inhibition in the cerebral cortex. The visual cortex is most commonly involved, but it can also occur in other areas, explaining the many different aura symptoms. A variety of environmental factors, including stress, lack of sleep and hormonal changes, can trigger the wave of cortical depression, particularly in someone with genetic predisposition. How the cortical depression causes headache is not completely clear, but vascular dilatation that accompanies the wave of depression and release of neuropeptides that trigger pain are likely explanations.

In Brief

Chronic back pain, abdominal pain and headache are by far the most common symptoms that bring patients to physicians. Although all three types of pain have potentially dangerous causes, in the vast majority of cases no medical cause can be identified, so-called medically unexplained symptoms. Imaging the back, abdomen or brain with CT or MRI is appropriate in a subset of patients, particularly when pain is acute and/or associated with "red flags," but it is rarely helpful for chronic isolated pain. Nonspecific incidental findings on imaging are an important cause for developing chronic pain via the nocebo effect. Depression, stress and inactivity are major risk factors for developing chronic low back pain, and regular exercise, including stretching and relaxation techniques, is key to successful management. Peptic ulcer disease nicely illustrates the complex interaction of biopsychosocial factors in the production of symptoms. Although infection with *H. pylori* and chronic use of NSAIDs cause gastrointestinal irritation, psychological stress and genetic variants can influence whether or not ulcers develop. Other environmental risk factors include smoking, alcohol use and obesity. In many ways, migraine is the prototypical psychophysiological disorder, with genetic underpinning overlapping anxiety and depression, symptoms associated with observable physiological changes in the brain, and stress a common trigger.

References

1. Engel GL. "Psychogenic" pain and the pain prone patient. Am J Med. 1959;26:916.
2. Rey R. The history of pain. Translated by Wallace LE, Cadden JA, Cadden SW. London: Harvard University Press; 1995.
3. Goody W. On the nature of pain. Brain. 1957;80:118–31.
4. Shorter E. From paralysis to fatigue: a history of psychosomatic illness in the modern era. New York: Free Press; 1992. p. 9.
5. Shorter E. From paralysis to fatigue: a history of psychosomatic illness in the modern era. New York: Free Press; 1992. p. 297.
6. Katz J, Rosenbloom BN, Fashler S. Chronic pain, psychopathology, and DSM-5 somatic symptom disorder. Can J Psychiatr. 2015;60:160–7.
7. Allan DB, Waddell G. An historical perspective on low back pain and disability. Acta Orthop Scand. 1989;60(Suppl 234):1–23.
8. McCullough D. The greater journey. Americans in Paris. New York: Simon and Schuster; 2011. p. 223–31.
9. Mitchell TG. Anti-slavery politics in antebellum and civil war America. Westport: Praeger; 2007. p. 95.

10. McCullough D. The greater journey. Americans in Paris, vol. 225. New York: Simon and Schuster; 2011.
11. McCullough D. The greater journey. Americans in Paris, vol. 230. New York: Simon and Schuster; 2011.
12. Erichsen JE. On railway and other injuries of the nervous system. Six lectures on certain obscure injuries of the nervous system commonly met with as a result of shock to the body received in collisions in railways. London: Walton & Maberly; 1866.
13. Allan DB, Waddell G. An historical perspective on low back pain and disability. Acta Orthop Scand. 1989;60(Suppl 234):13.
14. Osgood RB, Momson LB. The problem of the industrial lame back. Boston Med Surg J. 1924;191:381–91.
15. Buckley CW, Copeman WSC. In: Cope ZV, editor. History of the second world war: medicine and pathology. London: HMSO; 1952.
16. Mixter WJ, Barr JS. Rupture of the intervertebral disc with involvement of the spinal cord. N Engl J Med. 1934;211:210–4.
17. Baloh RW. Sciatica and chronic pain. New York: Springer; 2019.
18. Boden SD, Davis OD, Dina TS. Abnormal magnetic resonance scans of the lumbar spine in asymptomatic subjects. J Bone Joint Surg. 1990;3:403–8.
19. Reddi D, Curran N. Chronic pain after surgery: pathophysiology, risk factors and prevention. Postgrad Med J. 2014;90:222–7.
20. Walker BF, Muller R, Grant WD. Low back pain in Australian adults. Prevalence and associated disability. J Manipulative Physiol Ther. 2004;27:238–44.
21. Kent P, Mjøsund H, Petersen DHD. Does targeting manual therapy and/or exercise improve patient outcomes in nonspecific low back pain? BMC Med. 2010;8:22.
22. van Tulder M, Becker A, Bekkering T, et al. European guidelines for the management of acute nonspecific low back pain in primary care. Eur Spine J. 2006;15(Suppl 2):S169–91.
23. Baloh RW. Sciatica and chronic pain. New York: Springer; 2019. p. 47–56.
24. Hopayian K, Notley C. A systematic review of low back pain and sciatica patients' expectations and experiences of health care. Spine J. 2014;14:1769–80.
25. Bener A, Verjee M, Dafeeah EE, et al. Psychological factors: anxiety, depression, and somatization symptoms in low back pain patients. J Pain Res. 2013;6:95–101.
26. Denk F, McMahon SB, Tracey I. Pain vulnerability: a neurobiological perspective. Nat Neurosci. 2014;17:192–200.
27. Alzahrani H, Mackey M, Stamatakis E, et al. The association between physical activity and low back pain: a systematic review and metaanalysis of observational studies. Sci Rep. 2019;9:8244.
28. Steffens D, Maher CG, Pereira LSM, et al. Prevention of lowback pain, a systematic review and meta-analysis. JAMA Intern Med. 2016;176:199–208.
29. Park S-M, Kim H-J, Jang S, et al. Depression is closely associated with chronic low back pain in patients over 50 years of age. Spine. 2018;43:1281–8.
30. Toshinaga T, Matsudaira K, Sato H, Vietri J. The impact of depression among chronic low back pain patients in Japan. BCM Musculoskelet Disord. 2016;17:447.
31. Meier ML, Stämpfli P, Humphreys BK, et al. The impact of pain-related fear on neural pathways of pain modulation in chronic low back pain. Pain Rep. 2017;2:e601.
32. Eccleston C. Role of psychology in pain management. Br J Anaesth. 2001;87:144–52.
33. Bichat MFX. Recherches physiologiques sur la vie and la mort (Physiological researches upon life and death). Verviers: Gérard & Company; 1973; 1st ed. 1800.
34. Leriche R. La Chirurgie de la douleur (Surgery of pain). Paris: Masson; 1937.
35. Baloh RW. Sciatica and chronic pain. New York: Springer; 2019. p. 76.
36. Shorter E. From paralysis to fatigue: a history of psychosomatic illness in the modern era. New York: Free Press; 1992. p. 8–9.
37. Chey WD, Kurlander J, Eswaran S. Irritable bowel syndrome: a clinical review. JAMA. 2015;313:949–58.

38. Ladabaum U, Boyd E, Zhao WK. Diagnosis, comorbidities and management of irritable Bowel syndrome in patients in a large health maintenance organization. Clin Gastroenterol Hepatol. 2012;10:37–45.
39. Ballenger JC, Davidson JR, Lecrubier Y, Nutt DJ, Lydiard RB, Mayer EA, et al. Consensus statement on depression, anxiety, and functional gastrointestinal disorders. J Clin Psychiatry. 2001;62(suppl 8):48–51.
40. Gustafson J, Welling D. "No acid, no ulcer"—100 years later: a review of the history of peptic ulcer disease. J Am Coll Surg. 2010;210:110–6.
41. Beaumont W. Experiments and observations on the gastric juice and the physiology of digestion. Plattsburgh: F. P. Allen; 1833.
42. Schwarz K. Über penetrierende Magen- und jejunalgeschüre. Beitr Klin Chir. 1910;67:96–128.
43. Sippy BW. Gastric and duodenal ulcer. Medical cure by an efficient removal of gastric juice corrosion. JAMA. 1915;64:1625–30.
44. Warren RJ. Unidentified curbed bacilli on gastric epithelium in active chronic gastritis. Lancet. 1983;i:1273.
45. Marshall B. Unidentified curbed bacilli on gastric epithelium in active chronic gastritis [Reply]. Lancet. 1983;i:1273–5.
46. Marshall BJ, Armstrong JA, McGechie DB, et al. Attempt to fulfill Koch's postulates for pyloric Campylobacter. Med J Aust. 1985;142:436–9.
47. Sauerbaum S, Michetti P. Helicobacter pylori infection. N Engl J Med. 2002;347:1175–86.
48. Schoen RT, Vender RJ. Mechanisms of non-steroidal anti-inflammatory drug-induced gastric damage. Am J Med. 1989;86:449–58.
49. De Leest HT, Steen KS, Bloemena E, et al. Helicobacter pylori eradication in patients on long-term treatment with NSAIDs reduces the severity of gastritis: a randomized controlled trial. J Clin Gastroenterol. 2009;43:140–6.
50. Levenstein S, Rosenstock S, Jacobsen RK, Jorgensen T. Psychological stress increases risk for peptic ulcer, regardless of helicobacter pylori infection or use of nonsteroidal anti-inflammatory drugs. Clin Gastroenterol Hepatol. 2015;13:498–506.
51. Melinder C, Udumyan R, Hiyoshi A, et al. Decreased stress resilience in young men significantly increases the risk of subsequent peptic ulcer disease - a prospective study of 233,093 men in Sweden. Aliment Pharmacol Ther. 2015;41:1005–15.
52. Deding U, Ejlskov L, Grabas MPK, et al. Perceived stress as a risk factor for peptic ulcers: a register-based cohort study. BMC Gastroenterol. 2016;16:140–52.
53. Holtmann G, Armstrong D, Pöppel E, Bauerfeind A, Goebell H, Arnold R, et al. Influence of stress on the healing and relapse of duodenal ulcers. A prospective, multicenter trial of 2109 patients with recurrent duodenal ulceration treated with ranitidine. Scand J Gastroenterol. 1992;27:917–23.
54. Malaty HM, Graham DY, Isaksson E, et al. Are genetic influences on peptic ulcer dependent or independent of genetic influences for Helicobacter pylori infection. Arch Intern Med. 2000;160:105–9.
55. Levenstein S. The very model of a modern etiology: a biopsychosocial view of peptic ulcer. Psychosom Med. 2000;62:176–85.
56. Steiner TJ, Stovner LJ, Vos T, Jensen R, Katsarava Z. Migraine is first cause of disability in under 50s: will health politicians now take notice? J Headache Pain. 2018;19(1):17–21.
57. Steiner TJ, Stovner LJ, Vos T, Jensen R, Katsarava Z. Migraine is first cause of disability in under 50s: will health politicians now take notice? J Headache Pain. 2018;19(1):20.
58. Janke EA, Holroyd KA, Romanek K. Depression increases onset of tension-type headache following laboratory stress. Pain. 2004;111:230–8.
59. Sacks OW. Migraine: evolution of a common disorder. London: Farber and Farber; 1970. p. 29.
60. Sacks OW. Migraine: evolution of a common disorder. London: Farber and Farber; 1970. p. 21.
61. Sacks OW. Migraine: evolution of a common disorder. London: Farber and Farber; 1970. p. 24–5.
62. Sacks OW. Migraine: evolution of a common disorder. London: Farber and Farber; 1970. p. 26.
63. Sacks OW. Migraine: evolution of a common disorder. London: Farber and Farber; 1970. p. 82.

64. Sacks OW. Migraine: evolution of a common disorder. London: Farber and Farber; 1970. p. 114–5.
65. Todd J. The syndrome of Alice in wonderland. Can Med Assoc J. 1955;73:701–4.
66. Podoll K, Robinson D. Lewis Carroll's migraine experiences. Lancet. 1999;354:1366.
67. Weatherall MW. The migraine theories of Living and Latham: a reappraisal. Brain. 2012;135:2560–8.
68. Weatherall MW. The migraine theories of Living and Latham: a reappraisal. Brain. 2012;135:2567.
69. Liveing E. On megrim, sick-headache, and some allied disorders. A contribution to the pathology of nerve storms. London: J & A Churchill; 1873.
70. Latham PW. On nervous or sick-headache: its varieties and treatment. Cambridge: Deighton and Co; 1873.
71. Weatherall MW. The migraine theories of living and Latham: a reappraisal. Brain. 2012;135:2564.
72. Akkermans R. Historical profile: Harold G Wolff. Lancet Neurol. 2015;14:982–3.
73. Wolff H. Headache and other head pain. New York: Oxford University Press; 1948.
74. Goodell H. Thirty years of headache research in the laboratory of the late Dr. Harold G Wolff. Headache. 1967;6:158–71.
75. Lashley KS. Patterns of cerebral integration indicated by the scotomas of migraine. Arch Neurol Psychiatr. 1941;46:339.
76. Lashley KS. Patterns of cerebral integration indicated by the scotomas of migraine. Arch Neurol Psychiatr. 1941;46:332.
77. Leão AAP. Spreading depression of activity in the cerebral cortex. J Neurophysiol. 1944;7:359–90.
78. Leão AAP. Pial circulation and spreading depression of activity in the cerebral cortex. J Neurophysiol. 1944;7:391–6.
79. Anttila V, Wessman M, Kallela M, Palotie A. Genetics of migraine. Handb Clin Neurol. 2018;148:493–503.
80. Charles A, Brennan KC. Cortical spreading depression – new insight and persistent questions. Cephalalgia. 2009;29:1115–24.

Fibromyalgia and Chronic Fatigue Syndrome

8

> *The patient with FS [fibromyalgia syndrome], whether local or general, must accept that the cause of the ongoing symptoms does not relate to an extrinsic force, but rather it relates to factors under the control of the patient – to the patient's own psyche and pain system.*

> *Geoffrey Owen Littlejohn [1]*

Pain and fatigue are extremely common symptoms with both organic and psychogenic illnesses. The same brain pathways are activated and the symptoms feel the same regardless of the cause. In fact, most of the time organic and psychogenic factors are intertwined. As suggested in Chap. 1, why bother trying to make the distinction? To the detriment of patients and physicians, the debate regarding an organic versus psychogenic cause for fibromyalgia/chronic fatigue syndrome rages on with no clear winner in sight.

Pain but Much More

A 39-year-old woman had been living with daily chronic pain since her early 20s. The pain was more or less constant in her shoulders and neck, but it also could involve the arms and legs and torso on either side [2]. At times the pain was a burning sensation, while at other times it felt "like a tight cord was being pulled from my foot to my head." She had periods during which she was able to perform most normal activities, but at other times she spent days in bed so fatigued that it took all of her effort to sit on the edge of the bed. She had tried a wide variety of over-the-counter pain medications, none of which were very helpful. There were multiple tender points throughout her body that when touched caused her to flinch and pull

R. W. Baloh, *Medically Unexplained Symptoms*, https://doi.org/10.1007/978-3-030-59181-6_8

back. She would have the sensation that there must be a bruise on her shoulder or back but when examined there was no evidence of redness or swelling.

She had been bothered by headaches since age 12 that had features of tension-type headaches but at times were incapacitating with light sensitivity consistent with migraine. She had been sensitive to motion all of her life, with bouts of car sickness as a child and boat sickness as an adult, and over the past several years she developed a more or less continuous sensation of dizziness, which she described as a spinning inside of her head with no movement of the surround. Her motion sensitivity had become so severe that she could only ride in an automobile if she was the driver, and visual motion such as scrolling on a computer made her dizziness unbearable. She had problems with fatigue and insomnia since her teens, and over the past few years fatigue had increased to the point where it was as bothersome as her chronic pain. Her mother had been diagnosed with chronic fatigue syndrome in her early 30s, and she also had frequent headaches but had not been diagnosed with migraine. The patient saw a rheumatologist who indicated that she met the diagnostic criteria for fibromyalgia with typical tender points, and he planned on starting an antidepressant medication but first referred the patient for an opinion regarding her headaches and dizziness.

This woman illustrates the complexity of the fibromyalgia/chronic fatigue spectrum. Not only did she suffer from pain and fatigue, she also had headaches and dizziness and her symptoms waxed and waned with periods of incapacitation. Despite these severe symptoms, her examination and extensive testing were entirely normal. To suggest that someone could be "imagining" such a complex array of symptoms seems ludicrous, yet these patients are often told "the symptoms are all in your head."

Fibromyalgia

Fibromyalgia is a chronic pain syndrome characterized by generalized sensitivity to pain. For centuries, pain involving muscles and joints was called rheumatism (see Chap. 7). Scientific medicine was in its infancy, and archaic theories involving humors and vital forces still dominated the routine clinical practice of medicine. In the early nineteenth century, the Scottish physician William Balfour suggested that inflammation of the fibrous connective tissue of muscle was the cause of generalized muscle pain [3]. He was the first to describe focal muscle tenderness, tender points, where mild pressure caused pain and discomfort. Others suggested that the muscle pain resulted from hyperactive nerve endings or exudates from abnormal muscle vasculature. In the late nineteenth century, the American neurologist George Beard (see Chap. 3) included generalized pain along with fatigue and a variety of other somatic symptoms in his neurasthenia syndrome, which he attributed to the stress of modern living. At the beginning of the twentieth century, the famous English neurologist Sir William Gower described a new syndrome called fibrositis, which was characterized by spontaneous generalized pain, sensitivity to muscle compression, chronic fatigue and sleep disturbance, the basic features of modern-day fibromyalgia. Gower noted that the anti-inflammatory drug aspirin was of little use in treating the condition, and he recommended heat, massage, and local cocaine injections (for local anesthesia). During World Wars I and II, fibrositis was a common diagnosis among the soldiers, and considering the absence of inflammation and its association with stress and depression, some called it psychogenic rheumatism. The debate as to whether fibrositis (fibromyalgia) is an organic or psychogenic illness persists up to the present time.

Tender Points

The modern syndrome of fibromyalgia was shaped by a series of publications by the Canadian rheumatologist Hugh Smythe in the 1970s [4]. Smythe described fibromyalgia as a generalized pain syndrome associated with fatigue, sleep impairment, and emotional distress and he emphasized the importance of tender points for making the diagnosis. Investigators as far back as Balfour noted the presence of tender points but Smythe made them part of the diagnostic criteria. Tender points are pain sensitive areas typically where muscle tendons insert near a joint. Slight pressure in these areas causes pain so that the person flinches and pulls back. These tender points seem to be just below the skin and are scattered throughout the body in circumscribed areas in the neck, back, elbows, knees, chest and buttocks. Smythe initially required the presence of 12 tender points in 14 predetermined sites, whereas later criteria for fibromyalgia of the American College of Rheumatology required only 11 tender points in 18 predetermined sites. In essence, the presence of a high percentage of tender points was thought to be key to recognition and acceptance of the syndrome [5]. What do tender points represent and what are they telling us about the cause of fibromyalgia? Smythe suggested that the tender points were part of a deep tissue hyperalgesia (hypersensitivity to pain) and that they might originate from bone rather than muscle or tendons. But are tender points specific for and diagnostic of fibromyalgia? Here is where things get confusing. A study comparing 50 patients with fibromyalgia and 50 healthy normal subjects published in 1981 is frequently quoted as proof that tender points are specific for fibromyalgia [6]. The number of tender points in the patients with fibromyalgia was significantly greater than the number in the control subjects. But by definition patients with fibromyalgia must have tender points and in order for control subjects to be considered healthy they likely won't have tender points. Patients with fibromyalgia are aware of the locations of the expected tender points and the importance of the tender points in the diagnosis. Furthermore, several other diagnoses were more common in the patients with fibromyalgia than the healthy controls, including chronic fatigue syndrome, irritable bowel syndrome, primary dysmenorrhea, tension-type headaches and migraine headaches [7]. Others soon pointed out that there was an overlap between fibromyalgia and several other psychogenic illnesses, including panic disorder, depression, bulimia and obsessive compulsive disorder and that tender points were common in patients with these illnesses as well [8]. This set up a classic battle between the lumpers and the splitters. The splitters felt that fibromyalgia had a unique symptom profile with the specific finding of tender points, while the lumpers considered fibromyalgia to be part of a disease spectrum with overlapping symptoms and findings initially called "affective spectrum disorder." Even more bizarre, neurologists in Toronto, Canada pointed out an overlap in the location of fibromyalgia tender points and the location of what Charcot called hysterical zones, points on the body where pressure would trigger hysterical symptoms in his patients [9].

Central Sensitization to Pain

From the time of Gower's description, investigators largely considered fibromyalgia to be a disease of fibrous tissue and/or muscle. Abnormalities on muscle biopsy were reported, but the findings were non-specific and control specimens were largely absent. The only blinded electron microscopic study (the pathologist did not know the diagnosis in advance) compared biopsies from 21 patients with fibromyalgia and 11 healthy controls and found no difference in findings between the two groups [10]. Considering the absence of consistent pathology of fibrous tissue or muscle, investigators turned to the central nervous system for an explanation of fibromyalgia. The concept of "central sensitization" became popular because it could explain the sensitivity to stimuli in addition to pain, including motion, light, sound and smell and the high prevalence of stress, anxiety and depression with fibromyalgia [11]. Central sensitization could be influenced by a variety of factors, including psychological, hormonal and genetic, and the term was more acceptable to patients than affective spectrum disorder, which had psychiatric implications. Furthermore, studies showed that patients with fibromyalgia do have low pain thresholds to pressure, heat and cold. As discussed in Chap. 5, central sensitization to pain results from changes in the neurochemistry and connectivity in the spinal cord and brain pain pathways. Psychology is one of many factors that can change the chemistry and connectivity of the central nervous system pain pathways.

Repetitive Strain Injury (RSI)

In the late twentieth century, Australia experienced a major epidemic of work-related pain that cost the country hundreds of millions of dollars in lost work and in health and disability payments. In the late 1970s, there were sporadic reports of workers developing arm and neck pain, usually on one side, attributed to rapid and repetitive movements required in their occupations [12]. Although the pain was initially attributed to inflammation of muscles and tendons, examinations of the muscles and tendons were largely unremarkable, and some suggested there must be microscopic damage. As the syndrome became more frequent in the early 1980s, the descriptive term repetitive strain injury (RSI) became popular, and by the peak of the epidemic in the mid-1980s, mostly everyone in Australian knew about RSI [13]. Blue- and white-collar workers alike developed the pain, and remarkably it occurred in clusters, so that in some workplaces up to 30% of workers had RSI, whereas in other workplaces with identical jobs no workers developed RSI. Workers were told to be on the alert for early symptoms of RSI [14]. Any ache or pain might be an early indicator of the condition. Unions warned that the condition developed in a graded fashion and workers could rapidly pass from mild aches (stage 1) to severe intractable pain (stage 3), at which point there was no chance of cure. They also recommended that workers seek out doctors who were sympathetic to the diagnosis of RSI and would confirm that they were injured and could not return to work. Most of the affected workers did miss significant work time, and many applied for compensation. The syndrome even spread into the general community, and even a few schoolchildren presented to doctors with symptoms of RSI [15].

The pain would typically begin in the wrist or arm and then quickly spread to involve the shoulder, neck, chest wall and upper back [16]. The pain was described as a deep burning sensation often accompanied by muscle stiffness and tightness. Patients often reported numbness and tingling sensations, but there was no muscle wasting or other neurological findings. Fibromyalgia tender points were invariably present on the involved side but also commonly on the other side. A small percentage developed swelling and mottling of the involved extremity and a few exhibited typical features of causalgia (now called complex regional pain syndrome type II). The pain typically began on the dominant side, but in about half of the patients it spread to the opposite side, although it was usually less severe on that side. About 15% of patients developed generalized pain with involvement of the low back, buttocks and knees. Workers reported that the pain was made worse by changes in the weather, increased physical activity and emotional stress, and many could not return to work and even had difficulty performing routine household chores. Similar to fibromyalgia, many complained of sleep disturbances, headaches, chronic fatigue and mood disturbances. Once developed, the syndrome was relatively refractory to treatment. Prolonged rest, physical therapy, acupuncture, anti-inflammatory and analgesic drugs and antidepressant drugs provided little benefit, and the majority of patients reported slowly getting worse. Extensive diagnostic tests, including imaging the neck, electromyography, bone scans, screening blood studies including muscle enzymes and other standardized tests, were normal [17].

A rheumatologist from Melbourne, Australia, Geoffrey Littlejohn, proposed that RSI represented a regional form of fibromyalgia based on the presence of tender points and other features of fibromyalgia mentioned earlier [1]. Not surprisingly, there was immediate pushback from a variety of sources, including unions, lawyers and a large segment of the medical profession. Littlejohn suggested that much of this negative reaction was due to a general lack of knowledge about fibromyalgia in the lay and medical communities. To Littlejohn, fibromyalgia was a psychosomatic disorder in which central nervous system pain pathways became hypersensitive to pain (central sensitization). He felt that the descending pain modulatory system (DPMS) played a large role by changing the "setting" of the pain system at the spinal cord level (see Chap. 5). Mechanical injury might set off the condition by activating pain fibers from the area, but psychological factors served to amplify the pain and the long-term outcome was determined by the psyche and not the initial injury.

Others pointed out that RSI had many of the typical features of mass psychogenic illness. An index case with a work-related injury could serve as a template for the syndrome. Indecision and confusion displayed by the unions and health professionals caused fear and anxiety in the workers, accelerating the epidemic. The media played its usual role in amplifying the fear and anxiety with anecdotal reports of innocent people being injured at work and then developing long-term disability. Complicating matters even more, many of the journalists themselves developed the condition.

In addition to mass psychogenic illness, there was another elephant in the room – secondary gain. Once a patient was given a diagnosis of RSI, it confirmed their suspicion that they were injured at work and they then entered an entirely different arena of health care, the medicolegal system [18]. Here they would see a variety of medical specialists whose job was to provide a medicolegal opinion and not provide health care. Typically, medical specialists were chosen by the worker's lawyer based on their known advocacy for RSI and by the Workers Compensation Insurance Company, based on their known opposition to the concept of RSI. The different reports were then adjudicated in an adversarial system typical of workers compensation boards in many countries. Clearly, the vast majority of workers caught up in these medicolegal proceedings were not malingering with a primary goal of obtaining monetary gain. But once they believed they had a work-related injury and this was confirmed by the medical and insurance systems, they were in a bind – if they lost their pain, they lost their validity and disability payments. Complicating matters even further, at the time, if patients were considered disabled and unable to return to work, they were often given a lump sum payment. With regard to treatment, probably the worst thing these workers could do was to become sedentary and avoid exercise. But lawyers and physician advocates for RSI recommended rest and avoiding exercise. It was well known that insurance companies would secretly film workers, and catching them doing healthy exercise and sports could be used as evidence of malingering. The end result was avoidance of exercise and worsening of symptoms.

Littlejohn nicely summarized the workers dilemma when he wrote, "At the height of the epidemic an opinion given by a sound primary care physician was often disregarded by the patients, as they were often advised by colleagues to seek out doctors who would have a 'sympathetic' point of view toward their perceived injury. With persistence of symptoms the patient was often referred for another opinion to one of a variety of specialized physicians or surgeons. Such consultations would often attract a number of investigations before an opinion was sent back to the primary care doctor that the patient had been injured related to work practices. It is noted that the majority of specialists tended to either adopt the concept of RSI or reject it completely and assume the patient was malingering or hysterical. No alternative explanations for their pain were given. Multiple investigations and opinions led to confusion in the patient' s mind as to what exactly was wrong. This invariably reinforced the perception that they were severely injured, almost without any chance of recovery, and without help being offered by the medical profession, the traditional provider of care" [19].

It is worth pointing out that Littlejohn's diagnosis of fibromyalgia and a diagnosis of mass psychogenic illness in these workers were not that far apart, at least by current definitions of mass psychogenic illness – an epidemic disorder in which the psyche alters brain and body physiology. Although workers with RSI initially had localized symptoms, in most workers the symptomatic areas and the tender points spread to other parts of the body, and psychosocial stress was a major factor in the spread and prolongation of symptoms. Other probable epidemics of fibromyalgia-like disorders were described in soldiers during World Wars I and II and in association with other causes of musculoskeletal damage such as polio epidemics (discussed later in this chapter) and the Spanish toxic colza oil outbreak. A common thread running through all of these epidemics of fibromyalgia was an organic disease serving as a template for a psychosomatic disorder.

Chronic Fatigue Syndrome

Fatigue and exhaustion are universal symptoms experienced by everyone at some time in their life. Unlike pain there are no well-defined neural pathways for fatigue, and as a symptom fatigue is nonspecific and difficult to quantify. It is associated with a wide variety of illnesses, including cancer, inflammatory disorders such as rheumatoid arthritis, viral and bacterial infections, neurological disorders such as stroke and Parkinson disease and psychological disorders, including depression and anxiety [20]. Independent of the underlying cause, the symptom of fatigue has a major physical and social impact on patients and is a major cost to society in the form of medical expenses and lost work time. Fatigue is often separated into peripheral (muscle fatigue) and central (mental or emotional fatigue). Peripheral fatigue refers to the feeling of exhaustion after strenuous exercise, while central fatigue refers to a general lack of energy and difficulty concentrating that often brings patients to see a physician.

Surveys of otherwise healthy people show that between 25% and 40% of women and 15% and 30% of men complain of chronic fatigue, and the majority of them consider fatigue a major problem. Only a small percentage of these people are found to have a medical cause for their fatigue. In most it is thought to be psychogenic, the result of life stresses. It was the predominant symptom of Beard's neurasthenia. For centuries, fatigue and neurasthenia were synonymous. Since fatigue is usually associated with most medical illnesses, particularly infectious diseases, it is not surprising that many people attribute their fatigue to some yet to be identified illness. Fatigue is nearly always present in patients with fibromyalgia.

Epidemic and Sporadic Neuromyasthenia

In the 1920s and 1930s polio epidemics were common in Southern California, and in 1934 a particularly bad epidemic hit the Los Angeles area. At the height of the epidemic, the Los Angeles County General Hospital had 21 wards with 364 nurses caring for 724 patients, 360 of whom had polio. In this setting, 198 employees of the hospital, mostly nurses, came down with an ill-defined illness manifested by overwhelming fatigue and generalized muscle aching pain [21]. Understandably there was concern that the employees developed polio from contact with the patient, but they did not show the typical signs of polio and none showed the characteristic changes in samples of cerebrospinal fluid. Unlike the patients with polio, they had more sensory symptoms than motor symptoms with paresthesias (pins and needles sensations), muscle tenderness and generalized sensitivity to pain and they complained of insomnia, emotional upset and cognitive impairment. Furthermore, they were older than most polio patients, the course was milder, and none had permanent disability or died of the illness. The general consensus of public health officials was that the hospital employees suffered an unspecified viral illness. A few may have had mild polio, but there was no convincing evidence for any specific virus infection and some even raised the possibility of mass hysteria (mass psychogenic illness). Similar outbreaks occurred at multiple locations around the United States over the next 25 years, leading to a descriptive new diagnosis, epidemic neuromyasthenia [22]. The main symptoms were chronic fatigue, generalized muscle and joint pain, headaches and generalized irritability (remarkably similar to fibromyalgia). The cause was unknown, but it was assumed to be a virus or possibly an environmental toxin. Identical sporadic cases were also reported under the name of postinfectious neuromyasthenia. What was needed was a virus that could cause chronic fatigue and last for months and even years. At the time, viruses were thought to produce acute illnesses, not chronic illnesses.

Epstein-Barr Virus (EBV)

In 1961 English pathologist Michael Epstein attended a lecture on children's cancer seen in tropical Africa given by Denis Burkitt, a surgeon practicing in Uganda. Burkitt described an unusual cancer of the immune system in children that was endemic in Uganda, later to become known as Burkitt's lymphoma. Epstein, who was an expert electron microscopist, arranged for Burkitt to send a specimen of the tumor to Middlesex Hospital in London, where he teamed with a young virologist, Yvonne Barr, to identify viral particles in cultured cells from the tumor. Epstein and Barr published their findings in the English journal *Lancet* in 1964 and sent cell lines infected with the virus to Werner and Gertrude Henle, virologists who specialized in viral diagnostics at the Children's Hospital in Philadelphia [23]. The Henle's identified antibodies to the virus and, serendipitously, a technician working in their laboratory developed infectious mononucleosis and was found to have the same antibodies, establishing a link between the virus causing Burkitt's lymphoma and infectious mononucleosis ("mono") [24]. The virus, named the Epstein-Barr virus, or EBV, has been linked to other cancers, including stomach and nasopharyngeal cancer, and is ubiquitous in the general population. About half of young children and at least 90% of adults have antibodies in their serum, yet few ever had clinical symptoms. Interestingly, adolescents who have not been previously exposed are most likely to develop symptoms.

Infectious mononucleosis was known as an infectious disease that predominantly affects adolescents since the latter part of the nineteenth century. Even prior to discovery of the EB virus, there was clear evidence of involvement of the immune system with the diagnostic finding of characteristic enlarged white blood cells. The condition is transmitted by saliva; it is sometimes called the "kissing disease" of adolescents. The main symptom is severe chronic fatigue, but generalized pain and depression were also common. Clinical signs included swollen lymph glands, sore throat, mild fever and a swollen spleen. The overwhelming sense of lassitude typically lasted a few months, but in a small subset of patients, symptoms persist beyond 3 months and in a few they persist for years. The condition provided a potential template to explain anyone with severe chronic fatigue, and once a simple serological test for antibodies to EB virus was developed, the process of illness attribution soon followed. All that was needed was an outbreak with broadcasting to the general public.

In 1985 such an epidemic of chronic fatigue occurred in the small ski resort town of Incline Village on the Nevada side of Lake Tahoe. About 160 residents of the community developed an illness characterized by severe fatigue, frequent colds and problems with concentrating and memory (brain fog). The victims were predominantly well-educated, previously healthy, middle-aged women. A typical example was a 42-year-old woman who developed persistent extreme fatigue shortly after she ran a marathon in San Francisco. She initially showed gradual improvement, but then had a relapse so that she could no longer work as a business office manager. She noted that running even a mile would "put me in bed for a day and a half" [25]. Two local internal medicine physicians in practice together in Incline Village identified the first cases in the winter of 1985 and by the following spring they were diagnosing 15 new cases a week. Based on blood tests showing antibodies to EB virus in most of the patients and the similarity of the patient's symptoms to those of infectious mononucleosis, they proposed that the disorder was caused by EB virus, a type of late-onset infectious mononucleosis. They came to this conclusion even though infectious mononucleosis is not easily transmitted, no prior epidemics had been reported and, of course, nearly everyone has antibodies to the EB virus. Two investigators from the Centers for Disease Control (CDC) spent a few weeks in Incline Village and examined the clinical data but could not come to any definite conclusion. One of the local physicians developed a collaboration with Dr. Anthony Komaroff, an internist with a special interest in chronic fatigue at the Brigham and Women's Hospital in Boston, who concluded that the findings were "not all fabrication or hysteria or misinterpretation. I have guesses, but it is still a mystery" [25]. But the idea that chronic EB virus infection could cause chronic fatigue caught on with physicians and patient support groups who were looking for some organic explanation for the tens of thousands of Americans who suffered from chronic fatigue. The press called it the "Yuppie flu," a viral infection that predominantly affected professionals in high-stress occupations. The neurasthenia of the nineteenth century resurfaced as chronic EB viral infection.

Chronic Fatigue Immune Dysfunction Syndrome (CFIDS)

Gradually, the academic medical community began to question the evidence for chronic EB viral infection as the cause of chronic fatigue. Nearly everyone has been exposed to EB virus and has antibodies directed at EB virus in their serum, so how could the presence of serum antibodies be used as evidence for infection? Furthermore, researchers at the CDC found a poor correlation between patients with EB antibodies and patients with chronic fatigue [26]. They suggested a new name, chronic fatigue syndrome, to reflect the fact that the cause was unknown. Patient support groups refused to accept the proposed change in nomenclature and renamed their syndrome chronic fatigue immune dysfunction syndrome (CFIDS), emphasizing that it was a real disease of the immune system. At the time, virology and immunology were burgeoning new fields of medical science owing to discoveries in molecular biology and genetics. Reports in the lay press of possible new undetected viruses and altered immune function in patients with CFIDS provided new hope for an organic cause and a possible cure. One report suggested that a newly discovered herpes virus HHV-6 might be the cause of CFIDS. Others suggested that a yet to be identified retrovirus similar to the virus that causes AIDS could be the cause. Interleukins (ILs) are small signaling proteins produced by the immune system to stimulate the movement of immune cells towards sites of inflammation and infection [27]. ILs act on the brains of animals during infection and other inflammatory conditions, producing a response called sickness behavior, in which the animals appear extremely fatigued and withdraw from social interaction. Intravenous injection of IL-1 into humans causes extreme fatigue, fever and chills, and elevated IL-1 serum levels correlate with the degree of fatigue in patients with a variety of cancers. In patients with rheumatoid arthritis, administration of the IL-1 receptor blocker anakinra results in significant relief of the fatigue [28]. Unfortunately, anakinra does not appear to improve fatigue in patients with CFIDS, and studies in patients with CFIDS have yet to identify new viruses or immunological abnormalities not seen in the general public [29].

By 1990, epidemiologists estimated that at least a million Americans carried the diagnosis of CFIDS and as many as 5 million more had symptoms but were not yet diagnosed with the disorder. There were more than 400 CFIDS patient support groups, and the CDC was receiving more than a thousand calls per month about the syndrome. Patients communicated on-line about how to live with the disorder and how to obtain disability payments. New companies developed special clothing lines for patients with chronic fatigue and fibromyalgia, advertising comfortable, loosely fitting clothes with side zips that were easy to get in and out of.

Myalgic Encephalomyelitis (ME)

On the other side of the Atlantic Ocean, a similar scenario was playing out in England. In 1955, an outbreak of a strange illness manifested by profound lethargy, malaise, headache, dizziness, severe depression and emotional instability occurred in the Medical Staff of the Royal Free Hospital in London [30]. A resident doctor and a ward nurse were the first to become ill in July of 1955; by October, 292 staff members, including 149 nurses, were affected. Of the 292 affected, 265 were women. Despite the large number of staff admitted to the hospital, only a few hospital patients developed similar symptoms. The course of the illness varied, with some returning to normal within a month while others developed a chronic recurrent syndrome that persisted for years. Although a small subset had objective neurological findings such as numbness, weakness and eye movement abnormalities, neuropsychological symptoms predominated, including nightmares, hypersomnia, panic states and uncontrollable weeping. A few had mild fevers, but cerebrospinal fluid examination was consistently normal, and there were no other signs of systemic inflammation or infection. Several similar but smaller outbreaks occurred throughout England in the same year. Like in the Los Angeles County Hospital outbreak, an outbreak occurred at the Addington Hospital in Durban during a polio epidemic. Ninety-eight nurses developed extreme fatigue, malaise and a range of neurological symptoms, and 21 of them were unable to return to work after 3 years. Yet none showed objective findings of polio or any other viral illness.

These large outbreaks of ill-defined illnesses were initially diagnosed as encephalomyelitis, an inflammation of the brain and spinal cord presumably of viral origin, despite the lack of evidence for inflammation or viral infection. As in America, this diagnosis evolved as sporadic cases with identical symptoms were frequently seen in the general population. Since muscle pains were a prominent feature of the illness and the course was typically benign (no one died) the first iteration was benign myalgic (muscle pain) encephalomyelitis. In an editorial in the *Lancet* in 1956, after coining the term benign myalgic encephalomyelitis, the authors concluded "we believe that its characteristics are now sufficiently clear to differentiate it from poliomyelitis, epidemic myalgia, glandular fever, the forms of epidemic encephalitis already described and need it be said, hysteria" [31]. But patients were not comfortable with the prefix benign so it was dropped and the condition became known as myalgic encephalomyelitis, ME for short. Those following events on both sides of the Atlantic often used the cumbersome combined term myalgic encephalomyelitis/chronic fatigue syndrome or ME/CFS.

Mass Psychogenic Illness (Mass Hysteria)

A major shake-up in the ME/CFS community occurred in 1970, when London psychiatrists Colin McEvedy and A. W. Beard published two articles in the *British Medical Journal* suggesting that the epidemics of ME and CFS occurring in England and America were in fact, classical examples of epidemic hysteria or mass hysteria. In the first article, they focused on the outbreak at the Royal Free Hospital in London, reviewing in detail the complete records of all affected individuals [32]. First, they pointed out that the percentage of female hospital workers affected was more than 10 times higher than the percentage of male workers affected. How could this occur with an infectious disease? They then noted the predominance of subjective versus objective findings. Spontaneous pain was the most common symptom, followed by severe malaise; only a few had mild fever. On reviewing reported objective neurological signs, patients with flaccid paralysis had normal reflexes, and in those who reported sensory loss, the patterns of sensory loss often did not fit known neurological pathways, for example, a stocking/glove distribution or single or multiple extremities without involving the body. Clinical notes described fits in 10 of the 18 most severely affected individuals and in a few with detailed descriptions of the fits, the possibility of voluntary or hysterical fits was entertained. The patients thrashed about, clenched their teeth and held their breath. Diagnostic tests, including cerebrospinal fluid examinations, in 18 patients were consistently normal. They emphasized that encephalitis is a very serious disease, and one would expect abnormalities in the cerebrospinal fluid and at least a few deaths. Anticipating the likely backlash from patient groups and fellow physicians they concluded:

"Many people will feel that the diagnosis of hysteria is distasteful. This ought not to prevent its discussion, but perhaps makes it worthwhile to point out that the diagnosis of hysteria in its epidemic form is not a slur on either the individuals or the institution involved... the hysterical reaction is part of everyone's potential and can be elicited in any individual by the right set of circumstances" [33].

In their second paper, they reviewed the reports of 15 similar outbreaks of EM/CSF in Europe and the United States, including the 1934 Los Angeles County Hospital outbreak, and argued that these also represented psychosocial phenomena, a type of mass hysteria [34] (now called mass psychogenic illness).

They suggested a new name for future cases, myalgia nervosa. Not surprisingly, the expected backlash was quick and fierce. Patient groups rejected myalgia nervosa because of the obvious psychiatric implications, and physicians pointed out that a few patients had objective findings, including mild fever (although none with high fever), enlarged lymph glands, positive blood tests, such as elevated liver enzymes, and objective neurological findings, including facial and eye muscle weakness. Likely a small subset of patients in these outbreaks did have infectious disease, even possibly a mild viral encephalitis. As commonly occurs with mass psychogenic illness, the symptoms in a few index patients provide a template to shape the symptoms in the great majority with psychogenic symptoms [35].

Overlap with Depression and Other Psychogenic Illnesses

As noted several times in this chapter, there is overlap in symptoms between fibromyalgia and chronic fatigue syndrome, and many consider them a single syndrome with a spectrum of symptoms [36]. Indeed, the English diagnosis of myalgia encephalomyelitis (ME) combines both syndromes into a single disease entity. More than three-quarters of patients with ME suffer severe physical pain, and nearly half are bed-ridden due to extreme fatigue. Although the terms myalgia encephalomyelitis and neuromyasthenia suggest a possible peripheral muscle origin for chronic pain and fatigue, most investigators agree that the cause of ME/CFS is central, in the brain. Considering the overlap between fibromyalgia and ME/CFS, pain and fatigue likely share common brain mechanisms such as those described in Chap. 5 for chronic pain. Depression and chronic fatigue also greatly overlap, and physical fatigue and loss of energy are considered the hallmarks of depression. Patients with depression and chronic fatigue report difficulty concentrating and making decisions.

Simon Wessley, an English psychiatrist who had devoted his career to the study of chronic fatigue syndrome (CFS), decided to change directions and work in the field of military health after being the victim of constant harassment and threats from CFS patient support groups. In an interview with the London Times in 2011, he noted facetiously, "I now go to Iraq and Afganistan, where I feel a lot safer" [37]. Wessley wrote more than 500 research papers on CFS and developed a treatment regimen consisting of cognitive behavioral therapy and light exercise that helped some patients with this chronic disabling disorder return to normal functioning. What did Wessley do to deserve the wrath of so many people with CFS? He had the audacity to suggest that CFS had more in common with psychological disorders like depression than organic neuromuscular disorders like myasthenia gravis.

In one of his earliest and most quoted papers published in the *Journal of Neurology, Neurosurgery and Psychiatry* in 1989, Wessley, along with colleague R. Powell, compared symptoms of physical and mental fatigue in three groups of patients: (1) 47 patients with ME/CFS, (2) 33 patients with documented neuromuscular disorders like myasthenia gravis and (3) 26 patients with major depression [38]. In the paper, they called CFS chronic "post-viral" fatigue syndrome, even though they note that the condition was the same as what the Americans called CFS and that there was little evidence for a post-viral cause in their patients. Wessley later clarified that the name change for CFS in the paper was necessary in order for it to be published. They used a standardized questionnaire to assess physical fatigue by asking patients if they agreed with statements like "I feel weak," "I get tired easily" and "I need to rest more" and assess mental fatigue with statements like "I have problems with memory," I have problems concentrating" and "I have problems thinking clearly." The main finding in the study was that all three groups had about equal physical fatigue, but mental fatigue was limited mostly to the CFS and depression groups. In fact, these two groups had remarkable overlap. The few patients in the neuromuscular disorders group with mental fatigue also had depression. They concluded that CFS was a central disorder more like depression than a neuromuscular disorder. Not surprisingly, even though symptoms in the patients with CFS and depression were usually indistinguishable, when asked, patients with CFS thought they had a neurological disorder, while those with depression thought that they had a psychiatric disorder. The authors emphasized, "It is not our intention to adjudicate between the opposing views of physical or psychological aetiology. With the expanding knowledge concerning the biological basis of many psychological illnesses such a division becomes increasingly meaningless. However, both patients, and some doctors, continue to insist on such distinctions. It is instead our purpose to point out the serious consequences that result from this division. Not only will this lead to bias in research based on general hospital samples (as most has been), but it also suggests that many patients are being deprived of effective treatment" [39].

Why would this conclusion be so threatening to many patients with CFS? In the *Times* article Wessley suggested that the problem might simply be that he was a psychiatrist. "I think finally, fundamentally, it is that they cannot stomach the thought that this might be a, quote, 'psychiatric disorder'. By which they mean – not what I mean – 'it's imaginary', 'it doesn't exist', they are 'malingerers'." It matters what patients think about the cause and prognosis of their illness. Wessley continued, "Ultimately, a pessimistic illness perception can become a self-fulfilling prophecy of non-recovery. This group of CFS patients tends to view their symptoms as part of an overwhelming, mysterious, unexplainable disease that struck them out of the blue and from which they most likely will never recover" [37].

When asked years later whether his work had stood the test of time, Wessley responded, "I continued for the next decade to work on problems like CFS, and had some successes. We showed for example that it was not 'yuppie flu', and that it also was not untreatable. It wasn't plain sailing though, since it was impossible to get rid of the stigma of being a psychiatrist, which transferred itself to the patients. I found, and still find, that hard to accept, but it was a fact of life, and I became identified with the 'all in the mind' view of CFS, which was ironic since my interest in the condition was triggered by the fact that I did not think this was an imaginary or non-existent disorder, as many did at the time. Eventually I would move on academically, even though I continue to see CFS patients clinically." In the end, Wessley took a philosophical view of his conundrum, "Like it or not, CFS is not simply an illness, but a cultural phenomenon and metaphor for our times" [40].

Genetics of Fibromyalgia and Chronic Fatigue Syndrome

There is convincing evidence of heritability for both fibromyalgia and chronic fatigue syndrome and likely the two disorders share common genetic risk factors at least in part explaining the overlap in symptoms [41–43]. Families of patients with fibromyalgia and chronic fatigue syndrome consistently show a significantly increased incidence of both syndromes in first-degree relatives (parents, siblings and children) compared to spouses and other unrelated control groups. Even second- and third-degree relatives have a significant increase in the incidence of fibromyalgia and chronic fatigue syndrome, suggesting that the trait is inherited and not just due to a shared environment. Twin studies also have consistently shown a significantly higher incidence of fibromyalgia and chronic fatigue syndrome in monozygotic twins compared to dizygotic twins, confirming a small but definite genetic component to both disorders [44, 45]. Although numerous specific gene variants have been identified as possible risk factors for both syndromes, the size effect is small and the findings need to be replicated in multiple large population studies. A recent large genome-wide association study of 380,000 people in the United Kingdom Biobank with a diagnosis of multisite chronic pain identified 76 independent genetic variants significantly associated with chronic pain with a heritability of about 10% [46]. Genes for neurogenesis, synaptic plasticity and nervous system development were enriched in the gene-level association analysis. Interestingly there was a large overlap in the genetic associations with multisite chronic pain and the genetic associations of psychological disorders, particularly major depression.

Is it reasonable to consider fibromyalgia and chronic fatigue syndrome to be genetic diseases? Of course, the same question could be asked about other chronic pain syndromes discussed in Chap. 7, low back pain, irritable bowel syndrome and migraine. All of these disorders have compelling clinical evidence for a genetic underpinning. The answer to the question posed depends on one's definition of a genetic disease. There is a spectrum of genetic diseases from those caused by a single major genetic mutation to those caused by thousands of minor gene variants, any one of which alone would have a very low probability of causing disease. In between are diseases caused by a major mutation but require additional minor gene variations to determine whether and what type of symptoms occur. There clearly are chronic pain syndromes that are caused by a single major gene mutation but most cases of fibromyalgia, low back pain, irritable bowel syndrome and migraine are polygenetic and have environmental triggers that alter disease expression. These triggers include psychological, social and organic factors. Most would agree, however, that identifying genetic risk factors provides key insight into understanding disease mechanisms and developing effective treatments.

In Brief

Fibromyalgia is generally considered a pain disorder, but most patients have additional symptoms, most commonly fatigue, insomnia and dizziness. Chronic fatigue syndrome and fibromyalgia overlap in symptoms and are associated with a variety of psychophysiological disorders, including depression, anxiety and migraine. Patients with fibromyalgia have central sensitization to pain which can be traced to several factors including genetic variants, prior exposure to pain and stressful life events. Although many people believe that chronic fatigue syndrome is caused by a viral infection, post-viral activation of the immune system or primary immune system dysfunction, to date there is no convincing evidence for any of these disease mechanisms. Large outbreaks of chronic fatigue syndrome in the UK and USA had features consistent with mass psychogenic illness, including a marked female predominance and the lack of objective neurological and laboratory findings.

References

1. Littlejohn GO. Fibrositis/Fibromyalgia syndrome in the workplace. Rheum Dis Clin N Am. 1989;15:58.
2. Private patient of RWB, details changed to protect privacy.
3. Inanici F, Yunus MB. History of fibromyalgia: past to present. Curr Pain Headache Rep. 2004;8:369–78.
4. Smythe HA. Nonarticular rheumatism and psychogenic musculoskeletal syndromes. In: McCarty DJ, editor. Arthritis and allied conditions. 8th ed. Philadelphia: Lea & Febiger; 1972. p. 485–90.

5. Moldofsky H, Scarisbrick P, England R, Smythe H. Musculoskeletal symptoms and non-REM sleep disturbance in patients with "fibrositis syndrome" and healthy subjects. Psychosom Med. 1975;37:341–51.
6. Yunus M, Masi AT, Calabro JJ, Miller KA, Feigenbaum SL. Primary fibromyalgia (fibrositis): clinical study of 50 patients with matched controls. Semin Arthritis Rheum. 1981;11:51–1171.
7. Inanici F, Yunus MB. History of fibromyalgia: past to present. Curr Pain Headache Rep. 2004;8:373–4.
8. Hudson H, Pope HG. Fibromyalgia and psychopathology: is fibromyalgia a form of "affective spectrum disorder"? J Rheumatol Suppl. 1989;19:15.
9. Teive HA, Germiniani FM, Munhoz RP. Overlap between fibromyalgia tender points and Charcot's hysterical zones. Neurology. 2015;84:2096–7.
10. Yunus MB, Kalyan-Raman UP, Masi AT, Aldag JC. Electron microscopic studies of muscle biopsy in primary fibromyalgia syndrome: a controlled and blinded study. J Rheumatol. 1989;16:97–101.
11. Yunus MB. Central sensitivity syndrome: a new paradigm and group nosology for fibromyalgia and overlapping conditions, and the related issue of disease versus illness. Semin Arthritis Rheum. 2008;37:339–52.
12. Ferguson D. Repetition injury in process workers. Med J Aust. 1971;2:408–12.
13. Editorial. Repetition strain injury. Lancet. 1987;ii:316.
14. Browne CD, Nolan BM, Faithfull DK. Occupational repetition strain injuries: guidelines for diagnosis and management. Med J Aust. 1984;140:329–32.
15. Littlejohn GO. Fibrositis/Fibromyalgia syndrome in the workplace. Rheum Dis Clin N Am. 1989;15:46.
16. Littlejohn GO. Fibrositis/Fibromyalgia syndrome in the workplace. Rheum Dis Clin N Am. 1989;15:47–8.
17. Littlejohn GO. Fibrositis/Fibromyalgia syndrome in the workplace. Rheum Dis Clin N Am. 1989;15:48–53.
18. Littlejohn GO. Fibrositis/Fibromyalgia syndrome in the workplace. Rheum Dis Clin N Am. 1989;15:52–3.
19. Littlejohn GO. Fibrositis/Fibromyalgia syndrome in the workplace. Rheum Dis Clin North Am. 1989;15:49.
20. Norheim KB, Jonsson G, Omdal R. Biological mechanisms of chronic fatigue. Rheumatology (Oxford). 2011;50:1009–18.
21. Meals RW, Hauser VF, Bower AG. Poliomyelitis-the Los Angeles epidemic of 1934. Calif West Med. 1935;43:124–5.
22. Shorter E. From paralysis to fatigue: a history of psychosomatic illness in the modern era. New York: Free Press; 1992. p. 308.
23. Epstein MA, Barr YM. Cultivation in vitro of human lymphoblasts from Burkitt's malignant lymphoma. Lancet. 1964;i:252–3.
24. Henle G, Henle W, Diehl V. Relation of Burkitt's tumor-associated herpes-ytpe virus to infectious mononucleosis. Proc Natl Acad Sci U S A. 1968;59(1):94–101.
25. Steinbrook R. 160 victims at Lake Tahoe: chronic flu-like illness a medical mystery story. Los Angeles Times. 1986 June 7.
26. Holmes GP. Chronic fatigue syndrome: a working case definition. Ann Intern Med. 1988;108:387–9.
27. Norheim KB, Jonsson G, Omdal R. Biological mechanisms of chronic fatigue. Rheumatology (Oxford). 2011;50:1012–3.
28. Mertens M, Singh JA. Anakinra for rheumatoid arthritis: a systematic review. J Rheumatol. 2009;36:1118–25.
29. Roerink ME, Bredie SJH, Heijnen M, Dinarello CA, Knoop H, Van der Meer JWM. Cytokine inhibition in patients with chronic fatigue syndrome: a randomized study. Ann Intern Med. 2017;166:557–64.
30. The Medical Staff of the Royal Free Hospital. An outbreak of encephalomyelitis in the Royal Free Hospital group, London, in 1955. Br Med J. 1957;2:895–904.

31. Editorial. A new clinical entity. Lancet. 1956;i:789–90.
32. McEvedy CP, Beard AW. Royal Free epidemic of 1955: a reconsideration. Br Med J. 1970;1:7–11.
33. McEvedy CP, Beard AW. Royal Free epidemic of 1955: a reconsideration. Br Med J. 1970;1:10.
34. McEvedy CP, Beard AW. Concept of benign myalgic encephalomyelitis. Br Med J. 1970;1:11–5.
35. Shorter E. From paralysis to fatigue: a history of psychosomatic illness in the modern era. New York: Free Press; 1992. p. 310–1.
36. Wessely S. Chronic fatigue and myalgia syndromes. In: Sartorius N, et al., editors. Psychological disorders in general medical settings. Berne: Hogrefe and Huber; 1990. p. 82–97.
37. Marsh S. Interview with Professor Simon Wessely. The Times, 2011 August 6.
38. Wessely S, Powell R. Fatigue syndromes: a comparison of chronic "postviral" fatigue with neuromuscular and affective disorders. J Neurol Neurosurg Psychiatry. 1989;52:940–8.
39. Wessely S, Powell R. Fatigue syndromes: a comparison of chronic "postviral" fatigue with neuromuscular and affective disorders. J Neurol Neurosurg Psychiatry. 1989;52:946.
40. Wessely SC. Impact commentaries. The nature of fatigue: a comparison of chronic "postviral" fatigue with neuromuscular and affective disorders. J Neurol Neurosurg Psychiatry. 2012;83:5.
41. Arnold LM, Fan J, Russell IJ, et al. The fibromyalgia family study: a genome-wide linkage scan study. Arthritis Rheum. 2013;65:1122–8.
42. Mogil JS. Pain genetics: past, present and future. Trends Genet. 2012;28:258–66.
43. Albright F, Light K, Light A, et al. Evidence for a heritable predisposition of chronic fatigue syndrome. BMC Neurol. 2011;11:62.
44. Schur E, Afari N, Goldberg J, et al. Twin analyses of fatigue. Twin Res Hum Genet. 2007;10:729–33.
45. Mikkelsson M, Kaprio J, Salminen JJ, et al. Widespread pain among 11-year-old Finnish twin pairs. Arthritis Rheum. 2001;44:481–5.
46. Johnston KJA, Adams MJ, Nicholl BI, et al. Genome-wide association study of multisite chronic pain in UK Biobank. PLoS Genet. 2019;15:e1008164.

Chronic Dizziness

9

Some people become dizzy at the sight of a whirling wheel, or by gazing on the fluctuations of a river, if no steady objects are at the same time within the sphere of distinct vision.

Erasmus Darwin [1]

Dizziness is a nonspecific subjective symptom that can best be described as a feeling of disorientation or disequilibrium. It can take on many forms, from a light-headed near-faint sensation to an illusion of self or surround movement (vertigo), and it can result from a wide range of causes, including heart, inner ear, brain and psychosomatic disorders. Historically, dizziness has been a major part of the symptom complex of hysteria, neurasthenia, post-traumatic stress disorder, panic disorder, fibromyalgia and chronic fatigue syndrome.

Some dizziness sensations are highly suggestive of a psychogenic cause: floating outside of the body (depersonalization), constant brain fog with difficulty concentrating, spinning inside the head while the surround is perfectly still, sensations of falling yet having excellent balance and disorientation that just occurs in certain environmental circumstances, such as driving on a freeway and walking on a shiny floor, down a supermarket aisle or in crowded places [2]. Dizziness that is constant for months and even years is nearly always psychosomatic in origin. Psychogenic dizziness is highly prevalent in the general population and is one of the most common types of dizziness seen in dizziness clinics. In a study published in 1998, one in five people in a general practice community in London had experienced dizziness within the prior month [3]. Of these about half were handicapped by the dizziness and a third reported that the dizziness had been occurring for longer than 5 years. Nearly half of those who reported dizziness also reported anxiety and avoidance behavior along with other psychosomatic symptoms, and the number of psychosomatic symptoms correlated with the degree of handicap.

R. W. Baloh, *Medically Unexplained Symptoms*, https://doi.org/10.1007/978-3-030-59181-6_9

Anxiety and Dizziness

A 45-year-old man who had a longstanding history of anxiety and depression complained of dizziness dating back about 9 months [4]. His dizziness first started while driving on a Los Angeles freeway. He became lightheaded and had the sensation that his automobile was swaying. He squeezed the steering wheel tightly and had difficulty catching his breath but was able to make his way to the side of the freeway. There he noted that his heart was racing and he felt as though he might pass out. After sitting for about 20 min he was able to get back on the freeway and drive to his destination. He then avoided freeways and drove on surface streets. When he had to drive on a freeway 2 weeks later, he developed the same type of dizziness; this time he got off the freeway immediately and has not been back on a freeway since. His dizziness has gradually gotten worse, and he is unable to work. He stopped driving completely and avoids environments that aggravate the dizziness, such as supermarkets, elevators, and crowded shopping malls. Now he rarely leaves the house.

Driving on a freeway is a common trigger for psychogenic dizziness in Los Angeles. Patients report certain visual environments such as coming up over the brow of a hill or coming out from an underpass as being particularly provocative. Most will go on to experience chronic dizziness in other circumstances, but in some the dizziness occurs just when driving on a freeway and so they just avoid freeways and drive on surface streets. Most patients with freeway dizziness have obvious anxiety and panic attacks, with or without agoraphobia, and in some, the panic attacks are initially triggered by an episode of psychogenic dizziness. Anxiety disorders are the most prevalent psychiatric disorders in the general population, and, as noted earlier, anxiety can be primary or associated with other psychiatric and neurological conditions. Panic disorder is an extreme variety of anxiety disorder characterized by recurrent panic attacks with rapid onset and gradual resolution. Panic attacks are associated with the sudden onset of intense fear with four or more of the following symptoms: dizziness, palpitations, shaking, choking, chest pain, abdominal pain, depersonalization, fear of losing control, fear of dying, tingling of the extremities, hot or cold flashes and a feeling of suffocation [5]. Fear is a key factor in anxiety and panic attacks, and just the anticipation of a trigger for anxiety can initiate a panic attack. The end result is often irrational fear, avoidance behavior and agoraphobia.

The word anxiety has its roots in Greek and Roman words meaning suffocation, constriction and panic. In ancient Greece, Plato provided his interpretation of a panic attack in a woman with hysteria, "The uterus is an animal desirous of procreating children. When it remains unfruitful long periods beyond puberty, [it] gets disconnected and angry, begins to wander throughout the body, closing the air passages, impeding breathing, bringing about painful distress and causing a variety of associated diseases" [6]. The German neurologist Karl Friedrich Otto Westphal first described dizziness associated with agoraphobia (fear of the marketplace) in 1872 [7]. He reported three men who developed extreme fear of shopping in the open spaces of the town square. They developed dizziness, spatial disorientation and anxiety and had to be assisted by people passing by. Whether the dizziness and spatial disorientation triggered the anxiety or the anxiety caused the dizziness and disorientation was not clear. Around the same time in America, George Beard considered anxiety to be a major part of his neurasthenia syndrome and felt that anxiety could lead to morbid fears such as agoraphobia and anthrophobia (fear of society). Freud disagreed with Beard and separated anxiety from neurasthenia, calling the condition anxiety neurosis. He divided anxiety into acute (panic attacks) and chronic and described a wide range of somatic symptoms associated with anxiety including dizziness, cardiac palpitations, chest pain, sweating and shaking. He emphasized that anxiety symptoms were not "mentally determined" or removable by psychoanalysis but were the consequence of a disturbed chemical process [8]. Regardless, he still felt that abnormal childhood sexuality somehow contributed to the chemical abnormality. Like others before him, Freud considered agoraphobia to result from a patient's effort to avoid being struck by an anxiety attack in an unfamiliar circumstance where no help was available.

Near-Faint Dizziness and Fainting

Another type of dizziness commonly seen in patients with psychosomatic illness is near-faint dizziness, a lightheaded feeling as though one may black out. Nearly everyone has experienced this sensation at some time, particularly when jumping up rapidly after eating a large meal. The symptom results from a generalized decrease in blood flow to the brain due to a drop in blood pressure or alteration in heart rate. After a large meal, blood flow is preferentially directed to the gut for digestion, so there may be a brief drop in blood flow to the brain, particularly after jumping up. Anyone taking medication for high blood pressure is susceptible to brief lightheaded dizziness when standing, since the medication inhibits the rapid increase in blood pressure that normally occurs on standing. Many mechanisms can lead to a transient decrease in blood flow to the brain with psychosomatic illness. With acute anxiety, release of adrenalin and activation of the autonomic nervous system with the fight or flight response causes a redistribution of blood flow to muscles and heart at the expense of the brain (see Chap. 5). The sensation of smothering can lead to hyperventilation, decreasing the level of carbon dioxide (CO_2) in the blood, causing constriction of the arteries to the brain further restricting blood flow (see Chap. 6). Patients with psychogenic illness are particularly susceptible to vasovagal syncope, also called neurocardiogenic syncope or a common faint. This can happen to anyone, such as when seeing a nurse with a large hypodermic needle, but is particularly common in patients with heightened fear associated with psychosomatic illness. Fear can trigger a reflex decrease in pulse and dilation of peripheral blood vessels mediated by the vagus nerve (vasovagal syncope). The combination of slowing heart rate and decreased blood return to the heart due to pooling of blood in the pelvis and legs causes decreased blood flow to the brain and a near or actual faint.

Postural Orthostatic Tachycardia Syndrome (POTS)

Another common cause of near faint or fainting on standing, particularly in young women with anxiety, is POTS [2]. A 27-year-old woman with a long-standing diagnosis of chronic fatigue syndrome developed more recent lightheaded dizziness and faints when on her feet [4]. She fainted several times, and although she previously had markedly restricted activities due to severe fatigue, she now refused to leave the house. She could not stand for more than a few minutes because of severe lightheadedness. The symptom rapidly improved with sitting or lying down. Other associated symptoms in addition to the dizziness and fatigue included blurring and tunneling of vision, mental clouding, headache, heart palpitations and tremulousness. On examination, her pulse rate increased from 70 beats per minute while sitting to 120 when standing with little change in blood pressure. Typically, patients with near-faint dizziness on standing have a marked drop in blood pressure along with a slight increase in pulse rate. The diagnosis of POTS rests on the finding of a sustained increase in pulse rate on standing of more than 30 beats per minute without a significant drop in blood pressure. As with other causes of fainting, there are multiple possible predisposing factors for POTS, including blood loss, dehydration and chronic elevated levels of adrenalin in the blood. The single most common predisposing factor is deconditioning due to lack of exercise. In this case, the young woman had been spending much of her time in bed due to chronic fatigue syndrome. Lack of activity led to changes in the autonomic nervous system and hypothalamic-adrenal axis (see Chap. 5). Numerous studies have shown that the most effective treatment for POTS is a regular exercise program. By convincing her to gradually increase her exercise level, even though initially the dizziness was worse, she showed marked improvement within 3 months and had returned to most routine activities.

Dizziness and Mass Psychogenic Illness

Near-faint dizziness and fainting are among the most common symptoms reported in outbreaks of mass psychogenic illness. A typical example of an epidemic of fainting and near-fainting occurred in an all-girls school in Blackburn, England in 1965 and was well documented in the British Medical Journal in 1966 [9]. This outbreak is worth a detailed look because it illustrates many of the key features of epidemic psychogenic illness. On the afternoon of Thursday, October 7, 1965, the Blackburn Medical officer received an urgent call from the head-mistress of a girls' secondary school indicating that there was an epidemic of fainting among her students. "The girls were going down like ninepins" [9]. The day began innocently when one of the older girls fainted at morning assembly, followed by four more after assembly. The girls were asked to lie on the floor in the corridor, probably a mistake, since the dramatic appearance of the girls lying in the corridor likely affected what was to follow. By that afternoon 141 girls were complaining of dizziness and fainting along with other symptoms, including headache, shortness of breath, stomach pain, nausea and numbness and tingling of the face and extremities. Ambulances were called, and 85 of the sickest students were taken to hospital, where many were noted to be very anxious and hyperventilating. The school was closed until the following Monday, but when the girls returned to school an identical outbreak occurred leading to 54 more girls taken to hospital, and the school was again closed for the week. By the time the epidemic finally subsided 15 days after onset, about one-third of 589 girls at the school were affected. Of the girls taken to hospital, about half were released after initial examination, while the other half were hospitalized and underwent a range of diagnostic tests, including spinal fluid examination in nine without any abnormalities identified. The possibility of food contamination or a viral or bacterial infection was considered, but all tests for toxins and infection were negative. In hospital, several of the girls reported loss of sensation in a stocking/glove distribution or in areas of the body that did not fit a known nerve distribution, findings commonly seen in patients with psychogenic illness. Several displayed tetany, an involuntary contraction of muscles, a type of cramping, particularly of the hands. Both tingling and tetany are commonly associated with hyperventilation, since lowering of CO_2 in the blood reduces the level of ionized calcium and causes spontaneous firing of peripheral nerves.

After the epidemic was finally over, in retrospect, health officials pieced together the features of a classic case of mass psychogenic illness. Earlier in the year, an epidemic of polio in the town had received extensive coverage by the local press. Many canceled their holiday bookings in the town, and there were reports of truck drivers refusing to deliver goods to the "polio town." Further, the press provided detailed descriptions of the young polio victims, which had a magnified effect on the impressionable young school girls. On the day prior to the onset of the epidemic, the schoolgirls attended a Church of England ceremony that was under Royal patronage and, unfortunately, the Royalty was late; most of the girls were left standing outside of the building for nearly 3 hours. During this time, 20 students fainted or had to leave the line and lie down, and most of the girls reported feeling dizzy. One mistress noted that on the next morning bus to school there was "an air of excitement and a great deal of talk about fainting – exactly who had fainted and how many times" [10]. When the epidemic began, the local newspaper was full of speculation regarding cause of the "mysterious illness," which no doubt frightened the affected girls and their families. Overall, the symptoms were explained by fear and anxiety with associated hyperventilation due to the emotional tension. The fact that the symptoms persisted for a week or more in a small subset of hospitalized girls can be explained by recurrent anxiety or by actual learned behavior. Fortunately, in this case local health officials, including the hospital physicians, quickly recognized the outbreak as probably mass psychogenic illness and provided the necessary reassurance and nursing care that allowed the girls to gradually get better. Part of this process was to convince everyone that the girls were not malingering and that the initial responders were not inappropriate in their concern and alarm. In other similar school epidemics, unawareness of the diagnosis or inability of health officials and community leaders to convince affected students and their families of the psychogenic nature of the illness has led to chronic symptoms. This was particularly likely to occur when an unidentified toxic or infectious agent was thought to persist (based on rumor and media speculation), despite the lack of evidence for such an agent.

In his 2001 book on mass psychogenic illness, the New Zealand medical sociologist Robert Bartholomew identified 59 similar outbreaks of mass anxiety episodes in schools around the world between 1964 and 1996 that were documented in the press or in published medical reports [11]. Dizziness, fainting and overbreathing were the predominant symptoms in about one-third of the outbreaks, while headache, abdominal pain or screaming predominated in most of the remaining outbreaks. Twenty-three of the outbreaks occurred in the United States without any geographical pattern. In the book, Bartholomew included an article from the *New York Times* dated September 13, 1952 entitled "165 Girls Faint at Football Game; Mass Hysteria Grips Pep Squad." This article, which describes how these teenaged girls fainted at a Mississippi high school football game, not only provides a dramatic description of an episode of mass anxiety but also a glimpse of the football fanaticism in the southeast of the United States. The girls decked out in their "snappy" gold-trimmed black jackets and white skirts had paraded in town before the game, and they were so excited that they mistakenly marched onto the field at the end of the first quarter for their halftime performance. All were greatly embarrassed when the loudspeaker called them back to the sidelines. Then they began to faint. Onlookers noted "they fainted like flies." Every available ambulance in the area was called, and the loudspeaker asked for doctors in the stands. "But the game went on, with players dodging the ambulances." Five ambulances crossed the field at one time "like the race track at Indianapolis." By halftime of the football game, all the girls were in hospital and the second half resumed undisturbed.

One feature that stands out in these school outbreaks of psychosomatic illness is the marked female predominance. Of the outbreaks identified by Bartholomew, nearly all were exclusively girls or predominantly girls. Only a few were predominantly boys. Although the explanation for the female predilection is still debated, there are multiple factors, including biological, social and cultural, to be considered. Predisposing genetic factors and hormonal changes with puberty and menstruation have long been suggested as important factors, but so far no gender-specific biological marker has been associated with susceptibility to psychosomatic illness. Sociologists have largely dismissed the notion that females are biologically more susceptible to psychosomatic illness as sexist [12]. They point out that those who suggest biological susceptibility fail to take into account "gender socialization." In nearly all cultures, women are low in the power hierarchy and forced to develop submissive character traits that can lead to long-term emotional frustration. In many societies, girls attend separate schools if they are fortunate enough to be educated at all, and they are often exposed to social and psychological stressors. Girl schools in Malaysia and Central Africa are particularly prone to develop epidemics of psychogenic illness. Although most Western schools are gender-mixed without overt gender bias, girls are still expected to play the role of the "weaker sex" who can't control their emotions in public. The newspaper article on the fainting spells at the Mississippi football game nicely illustrates the concept of gender socialization.

Cultural beliefs, particularly in non-Western countries, often play a key role in epidemics of psychosomatic illness. For example, in many Asian countries folklore suggests that there is a contagious disease called *koro* that causes the penis to shrink in men and the breasts to shrink in women [13]. The condition is thought to result from an imbalance of the yin (female) and yang (male). Death is a possible outcome if proper treatment is not initiated (consumption of yang elements such as ginger and black pepper or placing clamps or string on the organ). Since the turn of the twentieth century, there have been several epidemics of fear of penis shrinking, particularly in young boys in school. The first report published in 1908 was by a French physician visiting China who described 20 boys at a school in Szechwan who had the perception that their penis was shrinking and disappearing into the abdomen. The boys developed extreme anxiety with typical associated symptoms, including near-faint dizziness, palpitations, sweating and insomnia. The French physician examined the last of the cases, and he could find no abnormalities, particularly no evidence that the boys' penises had shrunk. The boys' symptoms lasted as long as a week and spontaneously resolved. Many similar outbreaks of perceived penis shrinking involving thousands of people have been reported throughout the twentieth century in China, India, Thailand and Singapore.

In the early stages of a school outbreak, health officials must be cautious in attributing a psychogenic origin to the illness, because toxic and infectious causes may be present in a subset or possibly all the children. The investigation should be two-pronged: a search for organic causes with appropriate laboratory tests and a search for the typical features of mass psychogenic illness. Bartholomew listed the following features to look for [14]:

- Symptoms with no plausible organic cause
- Symptoms that are transient and benign
- Symptoms with rapid onset and recovery
- Occurrence in segregated group
- Presence of extraordinary anxiety
- Symptoms spread through sight, sound, or oral communication
- Spread occurs down the age scale, beginning in older or high-status students
- A preponderance of female participants near puberty and early adolescence

Managing these school outbreaks of psychosomatic illness is difficult and requires a concerted effort of health workers, school officials and community leaders. Not surprisingly, parents may initially have a hostile reaction: "How dare you suggest that my child is faking symptoms." "How could these terrible symptoms be psychological?" There are reports of physicians receiving threatening phone calls from angry parents. As with all psychosomatic symptoms, the parents must be reassured that the symptoms are real and that they are being taken seriously. School officials should focus on finding underlying psychosocial stressors and take proper steps to reduce or eliminate them. The risk of not thinking of or ignoring psychogenic features of these school epidemics is continued anxiety and chronic symptoms.

Persistent Postural Perceptual Dizziness (PPPD)

A 34-year-old man complained of chronic dizziness and sensations of falling dating back more than 3 years [4]. He described a variety of dizziness sensations from a "heavy headedness" and "brain fog" that was more or less constantly present to brief sensations of movement just lasting seconds. Any type of movement of either self or surround could trigger illusions of motion that persisted after the movement stopped. He had a constant feeling that he was swaying and might fall even when sitting in a chair. Despite these perceptions of movement and falling, he continued to work and carry on normal activities. He continued to play racket ball several times a week without any impairment in his performance. He was very uncomfortable in certain environments, such as going to a crowded mall or walking down a supermarket aisle with bright lights and shining floors. Although the symptoms made him anxious and caused panic-like sensations, he denied having anxiety or panic attacks prior to his dizziness.

This patient had seen many physicians for his symptoms, including five ENT physicians, and he underwent videonystagmography (VNG) testing on three separate occasions. Each of the studies was interpreted as showing nonspecific eye-tracking abnormalities, "a probable central vestibular disorder." Without boring the reader with extensive details of the testing, there are two broad categories of tests included in the VNG: tests of vestibular (inner ear) function and tests of eye tracking. Both have a wide range of normal responses, and the quality and accuracy of the recordings are highly dependent on the technician's training; the performance on the tests is dependent on the alertness and attention of the patient. Anxious patients tend to perform poorer on these tests than healthy controls, regardless of the patient's diagnosis. The most common abnormality identified on the tests is impaired eye tracking of a target moving back and forth on a screen in front of the patient. This is not a vestibular test but rather a nonspecific test of overall brain function. Yet abnormalities on this test are the most common reason for an interpretation of "central vestibular disorder." Based on the VNG test results, the patient was told he had a "vestibular disorder" and referred for vestibular rehabilitation therapy, which he performed on two separate occasions without clear benefit. He saw three different neurologists and underwent two MRIs of the brain and was told there were no abnormalities and that the dizziness must be coming from his inner ears. Not surprisingly the patient was frustrated with physicians and was confused about what they were telling him.

The type of dizziness experienced by this patient has been given many names over the years, including psychophysiological dizziness, supermarket syndrome, phobic postural vertigo, chronic subjective dizziness and most recently PPPD [15]. PPPD is defined as non-vertiginous dizziness and unsteadiness that lasts for 3 months or more without an identifiable organic cause [16]. Affected patients typically feel worse when they are on their feet, exposed to moving or complex visual surroundings and with active and passive head movement. The dizziness sensation is constant although it does vary in intensity with multiple possible triggers including stress, physical activity, environmental circumstances and emotional upset. But what is meant by non-vertiginous dizziness? The distinction between vertigo and non-vertiginous dizziness can be difficult. Vertigo is defined as an illusion of movement of the surroundings, usually an illusion of rotation. It can result from damage to the vestibular system anywhere from the inner ear motion receptors to the many nerve pathways that process the vestibular motion signals in the brain. But patients often have difficultly distinguishing whether they or the environment are moving. The sensation is bizarre and hard to interpret, so the description of the dizziness sensation alone is not reliable for distinguishing vestibular from psychogenic causes. Complicating matters further, PPPD can sometimes be set off by damage to the vestibular system. Vertigo can evolve into PPPD just as a painful injury can set the stage for fibromyalgia or an infection or inflammation for chronic fatigue syndrome. Furthermore, dizziness caused by vestibular disease has features in common with PPPD, particularly sensitivity to motion – either self or surround motion. Many patients with PPPD are convinced that they have a vestibular disorder based on comments from their physician and reports in the mass media.

The German neurologist Thomas Brandt initially called this condition phobic postural vertigo and noted that most of his patients with the disorder had an obsessional personality structure and typically had high standards of achievement and were highly ambitious, not unlike the personality traits that had been attributed to patients with neurasthenia and migraine [17]. Many of the patients had a prior history of other phobias and a family history of phobias. Anxiety and depression were also very common in his patients and their families. Brandt noted that despite the "vertigo," patients usually continued their daily activities with little difficulty. "A phobic patient can, for instance, conceal an attack of vertigo from his or her tennis partner on the way to the court, in spite of considerable inner tension, by stopping, supporting him- or herself and engaging the partner in unimportant conversation – and then go on to play a normal tournament match" [18]. He emphasized that this dissociation between a person's sensation of vertigo and their motor performance is rarely seen with vertigo due to vestibular damage.

In the early 2000s, psychiatrist Jeffrey Staab and colleagues at the Mayo Clinic in Rochester, Minnesota suggested that the sensation experienced by these patients was not vertigo but rather a non-vertiginous dizziness that could take on several forms: sensations of falling, sensitivity to self-motion, spinning in the head with no motion of the visual field, a rocking sensation not apparent to others and sensations that the floor was unstable [19]. They called the condition chronic subjective dizziness and postulated that the syndrome could occur purely as a psychosomatic illness in patients with anxiety and panic disorder or in the recovery phase of a known cause of vertigo, particularly if there was an underlying anxiety disorder. The basic idea of their theory was that dizziness associated with a precipitating event such as a panic attack or a sudden vestibular damage caused a re-ordering of the sensory hierarchy that the brain used for orientation and postural stability. The brain switched from relying on vestibular signals to relying on visual and somatosensory signals. As a result, patients inappropriately adopted risky strategies for maintaining orientation and posture such as hypervigilance and visual dependence. A vicious cycle developed whereby the dizziness increased anxiety and visual dependence, resulting in greater postural destabilization and disorientation. In 2010 Brandt, Staab and researchers from around the world met with the goal of developing a consensus for a name and diagnostic features of this dizziness syndrome [19]. The result was the term persistent postural perceptual dizziness (PPPD) and the characteristic features mentioned earlier. The World Health Organization included PPPD in its 2017 edition of the International Classification of Diseases.

In a recent large population-based study of PPPD symptoms in Wales, UK, there was a surprisingly high rate of PPPD symptoms preexisting in the general population [20]. Symptoms peaked in middle age and decreased with aging. Although symptoms were significantly correlated with migraine and anxiety, these factors explained only part of the variance. People with vestibular damage were excluded, so the symptoms could not be attributed to a prior vestibular disorder.

A popular explanation for PPPD symptoms is that anxious people become preoccupied with the conscious processing of balance and develop a heightened awareness of normally subconscious balance sensations [21, 22]. This results in a mismatch between perceived and actual postural movements, leading to the perception of unsteadiness. Environmental factors such as a vestibular disorder or a head injury could serve as a trigger for producing the full-blown PPPD syndrome, particularly in people with an underlying propensity.

Migrainous Dizziness

A 45-year-old woman with typical migraine headaches since age 13 began having severe bouts of dizziness, nausea and vomiting beginning in her early 40s [4]. During these spells, which could last for days, she stayed in bed and avoided any type of motion. She had had frequent bouts of carsickness as a child and boat sickness as a young adult, but she learned to avoid these spells by avoiding motion exposure. The bouts of motion sickness now occurred even without exposure to motion. Furthermore, her baseline sensitivity to motion markedly increased so that she could not ride in an automobile, even in the front seat, without developing severe motion sickness. She also became hypersensitive to visual motion, so that she had to curtail her work on a computer because scanning the screen would trigger a motion-sick sensation, and she dreaded shopping in malls where a lot of people were moving about. She noted that the spells were more likely to occur if she was under stress or if she had not had adequate sleep. Her mother and two siblings had migraine headaches and were also sensitive to motion with occasional car and boat sickness, but they did not have spontaneous attacks of motion sickness.

Patients with migraine experience a wide range of dizziness symptoms from chronic non-specific dizziness to extreme motion sensitivity to violent vertigo attacks [23]. By far the most common is sensitivity to motion, both self and surround motion, which occurs in about two-thirds of patients with migraine. Motion sensitivity typically begins in childhood with bouts of car sickness and persists throughout life, sometime with sudden worsening later in life. In some, the motion sickness is more incapacitating than the headaches. Many patients with migraine will report developing motion sickness during their headaches, and some will develop spontaneous bouts, as in this woman. Motion sickness is thought to result from a mismatch of sensory signals, particularly visual and vestibular signals. For example, when moving in a car or boat, the visual system sees the stationary surround of the car or boat while the inner ear vestibular system senses the motion of the car or boat. How this conflict causes motion sickness is poorly understood, but strategies that decrease the conflict such as driving the car or fixating on the horizon when on a boat can diminish the severity of motion sickness.

A condition called benign recurrent vertigo of childhood was first described in the early 1960s. A young child, often under the age of 4, suddenly becomes frightened, cries out, clings to the parent or staggers as though drunk, sweats profusely and vomits. Most have difficulty describing what they are experiencing, but some report a sensation of spinning. The attacks typically last minutes and then the child returns to play as though nothing had happened. The possibility that this might be a migraine-equivalent syndrome was suggested in the initial reports, but it wasn't until years later that follow-up reports documented that nearly all of these children developed typical migraine symptoms later in life [24]. Furthermore, no other cause was ever found. Other migraine-equivalent syndromes in children include recurrent bouts of abdominal pain (abdominal migraine), cyclical vomiting (without vertigo) and episodic vision distortion.

As with vertigo in children, benign recurrent vertigo in adults with normal hearing has been linked to migraine primarily by association – nearly all have a personal and family history of migraine – and no other cause can be found [25]. Furthermore, the vertigo attacks have many features in common with migraine headaches, including associated light and sound sensitivity, triggers such as stress and lack of sleep and sometimes response to migraine preventative medications. How migraine causes motion sensitivity, vertigo attacks or headaches is poorly understood. As we are beginning to identify the genetic defects that predispose to developing migraine (see Chap. 7), the common thread appears to be an increased excitability of nerve cells in the brain. Consistent with this observation, patients with migraine tend to be hypersensitive to all sensory stimuli, including light, sound, smell and motion – the prototypical central sensitization syndrome (see Chap. 5).

The picture is further complicated by the fact that anxiety, depression and fibromyalgia/chronic fatigue syndrome are much more common in patients and their families with migraine than in the general population. Anxiety-associated dizziness, near-faint sensations and faints and PPPD are all more common in patients with migraine than in the general population [26]. Understanding the mechanism of these different dizziness types in patients with migraine may provide a window into understanding psychosomatic dizziness and psychogenic illnesses in general.

Post-Concussion Dizziness

Dizziness is a common symptom of post-concussion syndrome, an ill-defined grouping of symptoms that occur after a concussion [27]. The presumption is that some type of brain injury occurred, even though in most cases no brain damage can be identified either on brain imaging or other laboratory tests. Some diagnostic criteria require a loss of consciousness, even if brief, while others require just a documented head injury. In addition to dizziness, symptoms include headache, insomnia, increased irritability, forgetfulness, obtuseness and loss of initiative. The dizziness is nearly always non-specific, and patients use such terms such as swimming in the head, lightheaded, floating, rocking and disoriented. It tends to be continuous for weeks to months. If vertigo, an illusion of motion, is present, then the possibility of associated inner ear damage should be considered. The most common cause of vertigo after a head injury is benign paroxysmal positional vertigo, a disorder that results when calcium carbonate particles attached to the otolith membrane in the inner ear are dislodged by the trauma and become trapped in one of the semicircular canals. Brief spinning spells (seconds) triggered by getting in and out of bed or turning in bed recur for weeks to months. This is an important type of dizziness to recognize, since it can be cured a simple positioning maneuver.

Post-concussion syndrome has long been at the center of a medical-legal debate. Is it a syndrome or not? How can it be diagnosed? How should patients be compensated? Proponents argue that it is a syndrome due to brain injury, even if subtle, and that it is a major cause of long-term disability and should be appropriately compensated. On the other hand, skeptics argue that it is not really a syndrome, because the symptoms are so variable and the same symptoms are extremely common in the general population, associated with a variety of psychosomatic illnesses. Research studies provide conflicting results, although most agree that psychosocial factors play a major role in determining severity and duration of symptoms. Not surprisingly, if there is clear evidence of brain damage on examination, immediately after the injury, symptoms tend to be more severe and prolonged [28]. However, the great majority of people have no evidence of brain damage, and there is a poor correlation between the type of head injury and the severity and duration of symptoms. Prolonged symptoms are better predicted by premorbid psychogenic illness than by the severity of head injury. Furthermore, there is no pattern to the combination of symptoms to support the concept of a post-concussion syndrome. One study in a trauma center found that post-injury symptoms were about the same in patients with head injuries or injuries to other parts of the body [29]. About two-thirds of patients had post-concussion–like symptoms, regardless of whether or not they had a head injury. A pre-injury history of anxiety disorder was a better predictor of symptoms than the type of injury. There is an overlap in symptoms between post-traumatic stress disorder and chronic post-concussion syndrome, and post-concussion symptoms are better correlated with traumatic stress than with head injury.

Dizziness and Fear of Falling in Older People

Dizziness is extremely common in older people. There are numerous causes, many of which have already been addressed in this chapter. The most common cause of vertigo is benign paroxysmal positional vertigo affecting about 1 in 5 people in the eighth decade. Benign paroxysmal positional vertigo is extremely frightening and can trigger panic attacks and fear-related restriction of activities. Calcium carbonate particles in the inner ear are less tightly bound with aging, so they are more easily dislodged. Older women with osteoporosis are particularly prone to developing the disorder. As noted in the prior section, there is a simple particle repositioning maneuver that cures the condition, but in some older people fear and anxiety persist, even after the positional vertigo subsides. Some even go on to develop typical PPPD. The clinical history is brief (less than a minute) spinning spells triggered by lying down, turning in bed or extending the head back to look up. Light-headed dizziness that only occurs when getting up from a lying or sitting position is a different condition usually due to drops in blood pressure, particularly in older people taking antihypertensive medication. Older people often use the term dizzy to describe a sensation of instability or imbalance when getting up to walk, yet they have no dizziness when sitting or lying down. Although there are many neurological disorders that can cause instability in older people, including a variety of degenerative and vascular disorders, anxiety and fear of falling invariably contribute to the disability.

Fear of falling alone, independent of any underlying medical condition, is a cause of disability and restricting activities in older people [30]. Since falls account for 90% of hip and wrist fractures and 60% of head injuries in older people, it is not surprising that people have concerns about falling. About a third of community-dwelling older people and more than half of people living in long-term care facilities fall at least once every year. More than half of community-dwelling older people report a fear of falling that correlates with social withdrawal and loss of independence. Older people who report fear of falling not only cut back with activities but also have diminished physical performance and are more likely to be anxious and depressed [31]. Depression is a major risk factor for developing fear of falling and falling. People with fear of falling use high-risk behaviors and strategies that actually make it more likely that they will fall. They become preoccupied with the mechanics of walking, focusing their attention on each step with little planning for future actions. For people to navigate through an environment containing obstacles such as a home with furniture and different floor surfaces, they must constantly search the environment for future impediments. Older people with fear of falling tend to become hypervigilant and direct gaze only one or two steps ahead with little planning for future steps [32]. This strategy leads to more frequent stepping errors and increased probability of falling. Physical therapy programs can be designed to help patients develop better strategies for dealing with fear of falling.

Sea Legs and Mal de Debarquement Syndrome

Sea travel on boats dates back as far as 60,000 years, whereas land travel on wheeled vehicles only about 6000 years. Traveling at sea requires a person to stabilize the body on a moving platform, a difficult task to accomplish that may take several days on board. The process of making the transition from land to sea has been called "getting your sea legs" and has been the subject of anecdotal speculations for centuries. The brain adapts to the continuous movement and the unstable platform using a combination of strategies. Sea travelers learn to increase the width of stance and body sway to improve postural stability and to decrease their reliance on vestibular signals and rely more on visual and somatosensory signals to maintain orientation. This process involves changes in brain chemistry and connections, just like all learning processes (see Chap. 5). When returning from a lengthy sea voyage, most people continue to use the "motion strategies" for a brief period of time until readaptation occurs, which explains the feeling of instability and persistent rocking that one experiences after landing, called sea legs or in French, mal de debarquement.

A 39-year-old woman returned from a cruise with her family 9 months earlier to find that the ground was rocking when she got off the ship [4]. She wasn't too concerned at first, but the symptom continued unabated for days and then weeks, and she felt unsteady on her feet ("like walking on a trampoline"), even though she was able to carry on most normal activities. The rocking sensation was present 24/7 whenever she was awake. The only time she felt better was when she was in motion, such as riding in an automobile, but after getting out of the automobile the rocking sensation transiently increased. Her only past medical history of note was a bout of postpartum depression after the birth of her second child and several panic attacks when she was in college. The continuous rocking was making her anxious, and she admitted she was becoming depressed. She had seen numerous physicians and had had numerous tests, including an MRI of the brain that were all normal. A neurologist noted that she was anxious and gave her diazepam (Valium), which provided some relief, but the medication made her feel "drugged," which she did not like. One of her main concerns was that doctors didn't seem to take her symptoms seriously.

Mal de debarquement syndrome (MdDS) is defined as a persistent feeling of rocking and imbalance like being on a ship [33]. It occurs after exposure to motion, most commonly in a ship, airplane, or automobile. Similar symptoms can sometimes be triggered by visual motion such as standing on a pier and watching a rough sea. Sometimes the symptoms develop spontaneously without any apparent trigger, in which case there is usually associated anxiety disorder or migraine [34]. As noted earlier, a constant rocking sensation can be a feature of PPPD. People with MdDS often report that the symptoms are least when they are preoccupied with daily activities and the symptoms are worst when they sitting quietly and thinking about the symptoms. Most people who have sailed on a ship have experienced the sensation of rocking after disembarking that lasts for minutes to hours. For the person with MdDS, though, this rocking sensation continues for months and even years. Uniquely, when a person with MdDS is in motion, such as in an automobile or back on a ship, the sensation of rocking temporarily abates. However, once the person leaves the vehicle and is again stationary, the feeling of rocking comes back and is often transiently worse. For unknown reasons, this disorder is more common in women than in men and is associated with anxiety disorder and migraine, particularly when spontaneous. While the exact mechanism of MdDS is unknown, the syndrome probably has something to do with maladaptation within brain vestibular and visual pathways, another type of central sensitization.

The motion one feels on a ship is complex. It is common, for example, for a person standing on the deck of the ship to experience combined roll to the right and the left and at the same time, heave up and down. One theory suggests that when a person is constantly in motion, the brain in some fashion learns to associate feelings of continuous motion with turning of the head from side to side, as when looking off the deck of a ship to search the water for dolphins or turning the head to look around the pool for the snack bar. When a ship passenger then returns to land and looks around to right and left, the brain recalls the previously learned association and produces a feeling of movement that mimics that which was present on the ship. In our modern world, the brain is constantly adapting to different motion experiences and usually it does so with little difficulty. As noted previously, sometimes it can take a while to make the adjustment, but eventually it does. However, with MdDS, for some reason, the brain becomes "stuck" in a constant motion mode.

Height Vertigo and Acrophobia

In many ways, height vertigo and acrophobia are typical psychophysiological disorders. When standing at heights, everyone slightly alters their behavior; about a third of people develop symptoms, including dizziness, and about 5% develop severe symptoms and avoidance behavior (a phobia). Descriptions of developing symptoms in high places and fear of height date back to antiquity, and no doubt our distant ancestors had good reason to fear heights, since a fall from a high place almost certainly meant death either from the fall or from the impaired mobility caused by the fall. There are both physiological and psychological factors in the development of height vertigo. We rely on our visual surround for postural stability, but when standing at heights and looking outward, we lose visual clues and our body begins to sway. Normally, the motion of nearby objects on the retina dampens the sway, but without nearby objects, the sway increases and can impair balance. The natural tendency is to try to get down onto the ground or floor to increase the sensory input from the hands and to provide a stable visual clue and then to get down from the height a fast as possible. A subset of susceptible people will develop a panic response and freeze so that they are unable to get down from the height and need to be rescued. This can lead to the development of avoidance behavior and acrophobia.

In Brief

Dizziness is a difficult symptom to evaluate because people use the term to describe such a wide range of abnormal sensations from intermittent light-headedness and spinning to constant brain fog and unsteadiness. Near faint dizziness is the most common somatic symptom reported by people during a panic attack and in outbreaks of mass psychogenic illness in school girls. PPPD is a psychophysiological syndrome associated with several other disorders including fibromyalgia/chronic fatigue syndrome, migraine, depression and anxiety disorder. People with PPPD have a constant sensation of disequilibrium even when sitting in a chair or walking on a flat surface and symptoms can be aggravated by shopping in a busy mall, walking down a supermarket aisle or entering a brightly lit room with a shiny floor. Despite the constant dizziness these people perform normally on balance testing. In addition to headaches, dizziness is an extremely common symptom in people with migraine with about two thirds of people reporting bouts of motion sickness often before headaches occur. Dizziness and associated fear of falling is a major cause of disability in older people independent of the many degenerative and vascular disorders common in that population. Rehab strategies aimed at relieving fear can improve mobility and decrease the risk of falls.

References

1. Darwin E. Zoonomia; or, the laws of organic life, vol. 1. 2nd ed. London: Johnson; 1796. p. 233.
2. Whitman GT, Baloh RW. Dizziness. Why you feel dizzy and what will help you feel better. Baltimore: Johns Hopkins University Press; 2018. p. 48–9.
3. Yardley L, Owen N, Nazareth I, Luxon L. Prevalence and presentation of dizziness in a general practice community sample of working age people. Br J Gen Pract. 1998;48:1131–5.
4. Private patient of RWB, details changed to protect privacy.
5. e Gurgel JDC, et al. Dizziness associated with panic disorder and agoraphobia: case report and literature review summary. Rev Bras Otorhinolaryngol 2007;73:569–572.
6. Nardi AE. Some notes on a historical perspective of panic disorder. J Bras Psiquiatr. 2006;55:155.
7. Stone MH. History of anxiety disorders. In: Stein DJ, Hollander E, editors. Textbook of anxiety disorders. Washington, DC: American Psychiatric Press. p. 3–11.
8. Nardi AE. Some notes on a historical perspective of panic disorder. J Bras Psiquiatr. 2006;55:157.
9. Moss PD, McEvedy CP. An epidemic of overbreathing among schoolgirls. Br Med J. 1966;2:1295–300.
10. Moss PD, McEvedy CP. An epidemic of overbreathing among schoolgirls. Br Med J. 1966;2:1299.
11. Bartholomew R. Little green men, meowing nuns and head-hunting panics. London: McFarland and Company; 2001. p. 27–54.
12. Bartholomew R. Little green men, meowing nuns and head-hunting panics. London: McFarland and Company; 2001. p. 34–5.
13. Bartholomew R. Little green men, meowing nuns and head-hunting panics. London: McFarland and Company; 2001. p. 33–4.
14. Bartholomew R. Little green men, meowing nuns and head-hunting panics. London: McFarland and Company; 2001. p. 46.
15. Dieterich M, Staab JP. Functional dizziness: from phobic postural vertigo and chronic subjective dizziness to persistent postural-perceptual dizziness. Curr Opin Neurol. 2017;30:107–13.
16. Staab JP, Eckhardt-Henn A, Horii A, et al. Diagnostic criteria for persistent postural-perceptual (PPPD): consensus document of the committee for the Classification of Vestibular Disorders of the Bárány Society. J Vestib Res. 2017;27:191–208.
17. Brandt T. Vertigo: its multisensory syndromes. London: Springer; 1991. p. 298–304.
18. Brandt T. Vertigo: its multisensory syndromes. London: Springer; 1991. p. 299.
19. Staab JP. Chronic dizziness: the interface between psychiatry and neuro-otology. Curr Opin Neurol. 2006;19:41–8.
20. Powell G, Derry-Sumner H, Rajenderkumar D, et al. Persistent postural perceptual dizziness is on a spectrum in the general population. Neurology. 2020;94:1929–38.
21. Guerraz M, Yardley L, Bertholon P, et al. Visual vertigo: symptom assessment, spatial orientation and postural control. Brain. 2001;124:1646–56.

22. Cousins S, Cutfield NJ, Kaski D, et al. Visual dependency and dizziness after vestibular neuritis. PLoS One. 2014;9:e105426.
23. Baloh RW. Neurotology of migraine. Headache. 1997;37:615–21.
24. Mira E. Benign paroxysmal vertigo of childhood: a long-term follow-up. Cephalalgia. 1994;14:458–60.
25. Slater R. Benign recurrent vertigo. J Neurol Neurosurg Psychiatry. 1979;42:363–7.
26. Eggers SD, Neff BA, Shepard NT, Staab JP. Comorbidities in vestibular migraine. J Vestib Res. 2014;24:387–95.
27. Baloh RW, Kerber KA. Baloh and Honrubia's clinical neurophysiology of the vestibular system. New York: Oxford University Press; 2011. p. 362–4.
28. Rutherford WH, Merrett JD, McDonald JR. Sequelae of concussion caused by minor head injuries. Lancet. 1977;1:1.
29. Meares S, Shores EA, Taylor AJ, et al. Mild traumatic brain injury does not predict acute post-concussion syndrome. J Neurol Neurosurg Psychiatry. 2008;79:300–6.
30. Deshpande N, Metter EJ, Bandinelli S, et al. Psychological, physical and sensory correlates of fear of falling and consequent activity restriction in the elderly: the InCHIANTI Study. Am J Phys Med Rehabil. 2008;87:354–62.
31. Murphy SL, Williams CS, Gill TM. Characteristics associated with fear of falling and activity restriction in community-living older persons. J Am Geriatr Soc. 2002;50:516–20.
32. Ellmers TJ, Cocks AJ, Young WR. Evidence of a link between fall-related anxiety and high-risk patterns of visual search in older adults during adaptive locomotion. J Gerontol A Biol Sci Med Sci. 2020;75:961–7.
33. Brown JJ, Baloh RW. Persistent mal de debarquement: a motion induced subjective disorder of balance. Am J Otolaryngol. 1987;8:219–22.
34. Cha YH, Brodsky J, Ishiyama G, Sabatti C, Baloh RW. Clinical features and associated syndromes of mal de debarquement. J Neurol. 2008;255:1938–044.

Treatment of Psychosomatic Symptoms 10

> *It may well be to the shareholder's advantage for pharmaceutical companies to promote medications for an ever-increasing array of human problems, but this in no way insures that these constitute improvements in health and medical care.*
>
> Peter Conrad [1]

For centuries, spiritual and medical healers have taken advantage of the most powerful treatment of all – reassurance. It works regardless of the cause of symptoms, but it is particularly effective with psychosomatic symptoms because fear and anxiety are often at the heart of the problem. The reassurance can be in the form of verbal support, an herbal compound, a pill, or a physical manipulation that the person believes will help. One might question the ethics of providing reassurance if the diagnosis and prognosis are unclear, but I would argue that there is no downside to being positive. Maximizing the positive and minimizing the negative should be at the heart of all medical treatments. There is a delicate balancing act, and one must be positive and provide reassurance while at the same time acknowledging uncertainties and providing accurate information about side effects of proposed treatments.

As suggested on multiple occasions in this book, the cause of psychosomatic symptoms can be traced to a combination of nature and nurture. In other words, environmental triggers initiate symptoms in a person with a vulnerable genetic and developmental background. Currently, we have limited understanding and ability to modify genes and no ability to change the past, but we can influence factors in the environment that trigger symptoms. Stress is the major driving force for the production of psychosomatic symptoms and fear, anxiety and depression are natural reactions to chronic stress. Everyone has stress at some time in life, but as Hans Selye noted, "*It is not stress that kills us, it is our reaction to it.*" So, we must first develop a strategy to manage stress in order to minimize psychosomatic symptoms. There

R. W. Baloh, *Medically Unexplained Symptoms*, https://doi.org/10.1007/978-3-030-59181-6_10

are a variety of ways to manage stress and improve psychosomatic symptoms, including lifestyle changes, mindfulness, cognitive strategies, medications and even more aggressive treatments such as electrical stimulation and surgery of the brain. Lifestyle changes, mindfulness and cognitive therapies are useful for treating all types of psychosomatic symptoms and overall are currently the most effective treatments.

Lifestyle Changes

If you were told that there is a highly effective treatment for psychosomatic symptoms without side effects that is rarely prescribed by doctors, you would naturally be skeptical. Furthermore, if you were told that the same treatment improves memory with aging and decreases the risk of developing heart disease, stroke and Alzheimer disease, you would likely say "no way." But there is such a "miracle" treatment – physical exercise, defined as a planned, structured, repetitive activity with the goal of improving physical fitness. Study after study has shown that regular physical exercise improves depression, anxiety, migraine, chronic back pain, and fibromyalgia/chronic fatigue syndrome [2–4]. When compared with drugs commonly used for psychogenic illness including major depression, exercise is equal or better. Furthermore, with exercise the patient is centrally involved in the treatment process, helping reverse negative thinking and the vicious cycle nature of psychosomatic symptoms. A common hurdle to overcome with physical exercise is that symptoms may feel worse when first starting exercise. One must get through this early worsening phase before reaping the long-term benefits of exercise.

Exercise and the Brain

Population studies show that people who exercise regularly live longer and have better mental health and fewer chronic diseases, including heart disease and stroke, than people who do not exercise [5]. On the other hand, stress and anxiety are risk factors for developing physical inactivity, and lack of exercise can lead to unhealthy behaviors such as smoking and overeating. Exercise changes brain chemistry and connectivity and in the long run decreases sensitivity to stress. The brain loves exercise. For example, exercise helps nerve cells eliminate potentially toxic waste products and activates endogenous endorphins that relieve pain and anxiety. Exercise improves neuroplasticity and neurogenesis in the hippocampus, reversing the shrinkage seen with anxiety and depression (see Chap. 5). Finally, exercise has a positive effect on areas of the brain involved in social behavior and has been effective in treating children with autism and adolescents with ADHD [6].

The key is to make exercise a part of one's daily routine. Any exercise is good, but vigorous exercise leading to sweating and increased pulse rate, for 30–40 min, 3 or 4 days a week, should be part of the exercise routine. Daily walks in the fresh air are ideal. Sports such as tennis, basketball, volleyball and rowing are excellent but are typically limited to a small subset of the population. Controlled muscle exercises such as yoga and tai chi combine mindfulness with exercise, so they are very good for stress management. Everyone can find some way to exercise. It is just a matter of setting priorities and making it part of the daily routine.

Sleep and Eating Habits

People with psychosomatic symptoms do best with a structured lifestyle including regular exercise, sleep and eating habits. In addition to exercise, they must allow enough time for sleep and eat regular meals and avoid fasting and binging. Eating a healthy, diverse diet makes sense, and people with anxiety should minimize intake of stimulants such as caffeine and chocolate. Sleep disorders are common in patients with psychosomatic illnesses, but regular use of sleeping pills is not the answer. With all sleeping pills, patients develop what is called tolerance and dependency, meaning that the medication becomes less effective with time and efforts to stop the medication lead to worsening of the sleep disorder. Occasional use of sleeping pills, no more than once or twice a week, is more acceptable. Melatonin, 3 to 7 mg, can be an alternative sleep aid and may also help with chronic pain. Stress and sleep impairment are interrelated, so managing stress improves sleep. That's why people who exercise regularly sleep better than people who are inactive.

Mindfulness

A major problem facing basic scientists and physicians in the late nineteenth century was the mind/body dilemma. Psychology by tradition had been a branch of philosophy, a discipline separate from the physical world. The mind was part of the soul, a supernatural entity that controlled the body through "vital forces" that moved through nerves to control muscles. The French philosopher Rene Descartes localized the soul to the pineal gland in the brain and compared vital forces to wind in a sail (see Chap. 2). However, with the development of scientific medicine in the latter half of the nineteenth century, there was a growing realization that diseases of the mind were diseases of the brain. On a daily basis, physicians saw how mind events were dependent on the state of brain function. A person's personality and behavior could be changed by a brain tumor or stroke. Scientists at the time predicted that newly developed research methods would eventually solve the "mind/brain problem" and make psychology obsolete, but we still have only limited understanding of the mind/brain interrelationship.

Consciousness can be thought of as the executive control system of the brain. Being conscious means being aware and able to experience oneself and the environment. It makes sense from an evolutionary point of view to have a single control system to adjudicate conflicting signals originating from different parts of the brain. Philosophers have long struggled with the concept of consciousness, even questioning whether it exists. What does it mean to be conscious? Are animals conscious and could future computers with artificial intelligence be conscious? From a medical point of view, consciousness is a clinical spectrum based on a person's level of arousal ranging from fully alert to comatose, unable to respond to any stimuli. Disorientation, delirium and stupor are different levels of impaired consciousness defined based on the degree of unresponsiveness. Neuroscientists continue to search for consciousness centers and pathways in the brain and have identified certain areas, such as the prefrontal cortex, that seem to be critical for executive functions. But patients with focal cortical damage, including damage to the prefrontal cortex (for example, after frontal lobotomy), have a sense of awareness and a sense of self and appear conscious to the average observer, despite changes in personality and altered behavior. Most likely consciousness is a distributed property of the brain, meaning it involves multiple redundant nerve pathways throughout the brain.

The idea that consciousness represents a continuous stream of mental events, one after the other, moving through the mind of a conscious person dates back to early Buddhist scriptures. The event could be a sensory experience, such as seeing or hearing something in the environment, a memory of something seen or heard in the past or an intention to look at or hear something. It can be a series of words or images. By focusing on the moment to moment conscious experience, Buddhists believe that one can achieve self-knowledge and wisdom, the basis of mindfulness. In his famous *Essay Concerning Human Understanding,* published in the late seventeenth century, the English philosopher and physician John Locke introduced the term *train of thought* to describe a train of ideas that continuously succeed one another in the understanding. The notion that consciousness represented a flow of ideas, one after another, was popular among philosophers in the eighteenth and nineteenth centuries. The American philosopher and psychologist William James preferred the terms "stream of thought" and "stream of consciousness" to emphasize that ideas melded together in a continuous stream rather than one event after another [7]. This metaphor even allowed for currents within the stream, representing subtleties within ideas. James felt that each idea, which he called "mind stuff," must be associated with a molecular state in the brain. Unfortunately, knowledge of how the brain works at a molecular level would require another century of investigation, so James could only speculate on the basic building blocks of consciousness. As discussed in Chap. 8, in the mid-twentieth century Hebb's "cell-assemblies," composed of loops of reverberating neural networks, provided a model to explain storage of memories and ideas. In the latter twentieth century, Kandel's work on neuronal synapses provide a molecular mechanism for the storage of memories and ideas. Still missing were the neural circuits that control the stream of consciousness and decide on what information to bring to awareness and what brain functions to leave on autopilot.

Stress and anxiety speed up the stream of consciousness so that one idea after another flows rapidly through the mind in chaotic fashion, making it difficult to focus on any one idea. We become preoccupied with the past and future and are unable to appreciate the present. Mindfulness is a way of focusing our mind on the present, where we are and what we are doing, so that we are not overwhelmed with what is going on around us. When we are aware of the present, we can assess our thoughts and feelings without judging them as good or bad. Mindfulness works by focusing attention on the body's internal rhythms to provide a sense of calm and relaxation. The goal is to live in the moment and not dwell on the past or anticipate the future. For example, a basic mindfulness technique is to sit in a chair with feet comfortably planted on the floor, arms relaxed at your side, head slightly tilted forward and feel your breathing in and out. When you notice that your mind is wandering, don't become concerned but just return it to your breathing sensation. The goal isn't to turn off your thoughts or feelings but to observe them and understand them. Mindfullness techniques can also be combined with exercise activities such as yoga and tai chi. Research studies have found that mindfulness can lower stress levels and improve overall health, protecting against depression and anxiety [8, 9].

Cognitive Behavioral Therapy

As noted in Chap. 4, behavioral therapy can be traced back to the work of B. F. Skinner in the mid-twentieth century. Behavioral therapy focuses on how the environment influences learned behavior and uses a wide variety of techniques to treat maladaptive behavior. For example, avoidance behavior can be treated by teaching people to substitute a new learned response for a maladaptive response by gradually moving up a hierarchy of fearful situations. Two ways this can be achieved are to have the person watch a video of people who use appropriate adaptive behaviors or to use virtual reality to provide realistic, computer-driven simulations of fearful situations. The increased arousal associated with stress can be treated with relaxation training where the person learns to reduce stress by tensing and relaxing muscles throughout the body. With counter conditioning, the person is taught to substitute a maladaptive behavior with a more relaxing behavior. Another key feature of behavioral therapy is the effort to quantify treatment outcome based on objective measurements. The patient and therapist agree on a "contract" outlining the nature of the therapy and expected outcome. In more recent times, behavioral therapy has evolved into so-called cognitive behavioral therapy (CBT), in which people use cognitive processes to control maladaptive behavior [10, 11]. People are taught to replace common errors in thinking, such as overemphasizing negatives and catastrophizing (the nocebo effect), with more productive thoughts, such as emphasizing positives and expecting good outcomes (the placebo effect) with the goal of improving their coping skills by challenging the way they think and react to stressful situations.

More recently, mindfulness and cognitive behavioral techniques have been combined into single treatments such as mindfulness-based cognitive therapy (MBCT) and acceptance commitment therapy (ACT) [12]. Since the goal of mindfulness is to teach people to focus on the present and accept thoughts and feelings without judgment, mindfulness makes it easier to let go of negative thoughts and emotions and replace them with positive thoughts and emotions, the goal of CBT. Studies of MBCT and ACT and other acceptance- and mindfulness-based approaches suggest that increased focus on the present moment allows people to better recognize thoughts and emotions that need to be changed and provides better insights into how to make the changes and switch attention from one stimulus to another.

Internet-Directed Therapy

Major limitations of one-on-one psychotherapy are the cost and lack of availability. Treatment sessions are time-consuming and costly, and most people don't have access to these treatments. One possible solution is internet-directed therapy that can be made widely available to the general public. At present, most internet treatments are managed by a therapist who either interacts with the patient on-line or reviews the material completed on-line and provides feedback to the patient (a type of group therapy) [13]. Both mindfulness and CBT programs are readily available on the internet and many are available through apps on a smartphone. Although it is still the wild west with regard to evaluating the success of different internet treatment programs, studies suggest that therapist-guided programs are generally more effective than self-guided programs, although self-guided programs are more effective than no therapy. Of course, cost effectiveness and safety need to be taken into consideration, and different psychogenic illnesses require different treatment approaches. A major potential advantage of internet-based psychological interventions is in the design and implementation of controlled treatment trials. It has always been extremely difficult to objectively compare the effectiveness of different individual psychotherapies. The costs are high and the numbers are small, and appropriate control groups are usually not available. With internet interventions, large sample sizes can be studied in a relatively short period of time. Recruitment is not geographically confined, and therapists can be much more efficient with their time by using prepared on-line material. This allows for a multifactorial study design comparing different treatment modalities delivered in different ways. For example, mindfulness, CBT and a combination of the two could be compared in a scheduled or on-request format. Blinded random assignment of people to different treatment groups is easily accomplished with internet-based therapies. To date, internet-based psychotherapies have mainly been used to treat patients with generalized anxiety and depression, since these disorders are highly prevalent in the general population and there is a general consensus that at least some people do benefit from internet treatment [14, 15].

Drug Treatments

Currently, no drugs have been developed that cure psychosomatic illness. A variety of drugs are used to treat symptoms, but the relative effectiveness of these drugs for improving psychosomatic symptoms is largely untested. Furthermore, all of the drugs have side effects and whether the benefits exceed the risks is not always clear. Current drug treatments for psychogenic illnesses can be divided into four broad categories based on the presumed mechanism of function: drugs that increase monoamine neurotransmitters (serotonin, noradrenalin and dopamine), drugs that decrease excitatory neurotransmission, drugs that enhance neuroplasticity and neurogenesis and drugs that activate the endocannibinoid system (see Chap. 5). Although this breakdown of drugs based on the presumed mechanism of action is useful for didactic purposes, it is important to keep in mind that most of these drugs have multiple mechanisms of action and we still don't know which of these mechanisms or combination of mechanisms is responsible for benefit when it occurs. Most of these drugs were initially developed to treat depression and anxiety and then tried in patients with other psychosomatic illnesses with varying success. The majority of patients with psychosomatic symptoms suffer from depression and anxiety, commonly both, and depression and anxiety are the causes of many psychosomatic symptoms. Many consider anxiety and depression to be two sides of the same coin, meaning they share some common underlying mechanisms. They can occur completely separate, however.

Although each drug used for treating psychogenic illness has unique effects and side effects, there are some common features that are important to understand before considering a treatment trial. First, these drugs are not penicillin, a drug that cures an infectious disease with a relatively brief course of treatment. None of the drugs cure the underlying disease process as it is currently understood, and most require long-term treatment (months to years) for maximum benefit. Patients must understand these limitations so that they do not give up on the medication prematurely. Symptoms often become worse before they become better. In particular, people with anxiety tend not to tolerate side effects and worsening of baseline symptoms and are more likely to prematurely stop the medication. All of the drugs have multiple effects on neurotransmitters in the brain, and many of these effects have nothing to do with the underlying disease process, so-called off-target effects. Even drugs with a name that implies a highly specific mechanism such as selective serotonin and noradrenalin reuptake inhibitors have multiple off-target effects. As a rule, it is always best to start with small doses and then gradually increase the dose depending on the response and associated side effects. How does one decide when to stop a medication that is effective? Unfortunately, this is an area where there are few data from controlled treatment trials, since most studies do not go beyond a year. As a general rule, it is best to gradually taper off the medication over several weeks and even slower, if symptoms recur. Finally, many of these drugs can have adverse interactions with other drugs that patients may be taking, and there may be additive effects such as drowsiness and constipation when multiple drugs with similar mechanisms are used.

Drugs that Increase Brain Monoamines (Antidepressants)

The story of how these drugs were discovered provides a good glimpse into the chaotic world of drug development in the twentieth century. The story begins with two chance clinical observations in the 1950s that ultimately led to the working hypothesis that depression was caused by depletion of monoamine neurotransmitters (serotonin, noradrenalin and dopamine) in the brain [16]. Tuberculosis was the plague of modern civilization so there was great excitement in the mid-twentieth century, when scientists reported that the drug, isoniazid, markedly cut the death rate. In the process of trying to improve the drug's effectiveness, chemists developed a derivative of isoniazid called iproniazid. When iproniazid was given to patients with tuberculosis some of them reported that the drug produced euphoria with overall improved mood. This observation led to trials of iproniazid in patients with clinical depression and reports of improvement in a high percentage of patients. Iproniazide was shown to be a potent monoamine oxidase (MAO) inhibitor, a key enzyme in the brain to break down of monoamines, so by blocking the enzyme the level of monoamines increased at the synaptic junctions. The second chance observation was that the drug reserpine, used to treat high blood pressure, caused depression in some patients. An extract from the plant Rauwolfia serpentine, reserpine was found to block a key monoamine transporter in the brain, leading to a depletion of brain monoamines. So, drugs that increased brain monoamines improved depression, while drugs that decreased monoamines caused depression, leading to the monoamine/depression hypothesis.

Unfortunately, the MAO inhibitor iproniazid had dangerous side effects, including frightening episodes of increased heart rate, hypertension and sweating, so despite the benefit for depression, it was eventually removed from the market. Other less toxic MAO inhibitors were developed, but because of side effects and interactions with other drugs, they were never widely prescribed in the United States. Another drug found by chance to be useful for depression in the late 1950s was the tricyclic amine, imipramine. Chemists modified the newly discovered antipsychotic drug promethazine to produce imipramine and gave it to a psychiatrist, Dr. Roland Kuhn, to test in psychiatric patients. Kuhn reported that it was a miracle drug in some patients with depression and overall it had relatively few side effects, at least compared to MAO inhibitors [17]. The mechanism of action of imipramine was unknown when it was first discovered but later it was shown to block both the noradrenalin and serotonin reuptake transporters, leading to increased levels of these monoamine neurotransmitters in the brain. However, imipramine (Tofranil) and several other tricyclic amines that were synthetized shortly after – amitriptyline (Elavil), nortriptyline (Pamelor), desipramine (Norpramin) – were found to have multiple off-target effects, including blocking several other neurotransmitter receptors and producing a range of side effects including dizziness, dryness of mucous membranes, drowsiness, increased appetite with weight gain and even mild memory impairment. Despite these potential side effects, tricyclic amine antidepressant drugs are still widely used for depression and a variety of other psychogenic illnesses, including generalized anxiety, chronic pain, migraine, fibromyalgia/chronic fatigue syndrome and panic disorder. Overall, the different tricyclic amines have similar therapeutic and side effects, although individual patients may respond differently to different drugs. Amitriptyline tends to be more sedating than the other tricyclic drugs, so it can be useful in patients who have sleep impairment as part of their psychogenic illness.

In the late 1960s, pharmaceutical companies focused their attention on the mono-amine serotonin after a postmortem study of depressed patients who committed suicide found significantly decreased levels of serotonin in their brains [18]. This led in the synthesis of a new drug, fluoxetine, shown to be a highly selective blocker of the serotonin reuptake transporter with relatively little effect on the noradrenalin reuptake transporter. Fluoxetine (Prozac) was finally approved by the FDA in 1987 and immediately touted as the new wonder drug for depression [19]. Synthesis of several other selective serotonin reuptake inhibitors followed, including paroxetine (Paxil), citalopram (Celexa), escitalopram (Lexapro) and sertraline (Zoloft), but in time, just as with the earlier antidepressant drugs, problems arose. A significant number of depressed patients do not respond to these drugs, and there are off-target effects, most commonly nausea, insomnia and sexual dysfunction. In another approach, pharmaceutical companies searched for drugs that blocked both serotonin and noradrenalin reuptake transporters but without the many off-target effects associated with the tricyclic amines. The result was the development and marketing of the selective serotonin and noradrenalin reuptake inhibitor, venlafaxine (Effexor) in the 1990s, followed by duloxetine (Cymbalta) and milnacipram (Savella) at the turn of the twenty-first century. As with initial marketing of Prozac, there was great enthusiasm for these drugs, but with time clinical trials have shown no convincing difference in the effectiveness of the two classes of drugs for treating depression and anxiety, and both have similar side effects [20]. As with the tricyclic amines, both classes of reuptake inhibitors have been used for a wide range of other psychogenic illnesses in addition to depression and anxiety (chronic pain, fibromyalgia/chronic fatigue syndrome, persistent postural perceptual dizziness etc.), but there is little evidence that one class of drugs is any better than the other. As suggested in Chap. 6, some have questioned whether any of these drugs are significantly better than placebo for treating depression, and most would agree that the monoamine hypotheses is at best an oversimplification. Monoamine levels in the brain are related to psychogenic illness but not the cause.

Drugs that Decrease Excitatory (Glutamate) Transmission

As noted in Chap. 5, glutamate is the main excitatory neurotransmitter in the brain, released at more than half of all synapses. When an electrical impulse reaches the nerve terminal (synapse), it triggers the release of small packets of glutamate that cross the synapse to activate receptors on the target neurons. This causes the target neurons to fire and pass the signal on to other neurons. Repetitive firing at synapses (Hepp's synapses) can lead to central sensitization (a form of neuroplasticity). There are hundreds of proteins involved in packaging and release of glutamate, producing and maintaining the glutamate receptors and degrading and transporting glutamate at the synapse. Slight genetic variations in the genes that code for these proteins can predispose to developing central sensitization, and all of these proteins are potential targets for new drugs that decrease excitatory transmission. Although central sensitization with chronic pain is best known (see Chap. 5), it is also associated with a variety of psychogenic illnesses, including anxiety and depression. Central sensitization of excitatory transmission in parts of the hippocampus and amygdala is a feature of anxiety and depression. Patients with major depression have elevated glutamate levels in the blood and spinal fluid, and monoamine-based antidepressant drugs reduce these levels of glutamate [17]. Drugs that increase brain monoamines may in fact work by modulating glutamate transmission and decreasing central sensitization.

Antiepileptic Drugs

A variety of antiepileptic drugs known to inhibit excitatory glutamate transmission have been used either as an adjunct or primary treatment of depression, anxiety and chronic pain. The most commonly used drugs include carbamazepine (Tegretol), oxcarbazepine (Trileptal), lamotrigine (Lamictal), Levetiracetam (Keppra) and the gabapentinoids, gabapentin (Neurontin) and pregabalin (Lyrica). These drugs work by blocking ion channels such as sodium and calcium channels that allow ions to enter the nerve cell and trigger the release of glutamate at the synapse. Because of the generalized action of the drugs, most have potentially serious side effects and interactions with other drugs. They are mostly used for serious cases of depression that fail treatment with more traditional antidepressant drugs. An exception to this rule, the gabapentinoids have relatively few side effects and essentially no significant drug interactions. In addition to blocking a subunit of a calcium channel critical for excitatory transmission, the gabapentinoids, particularly pregabalin, enhance GABA inhibitory neurotransmission, so there is a combined effect of decreasing excitatory neurotransmission and increasing inhibitory neurotransmission. Although the actions of gabapentin and pregabalin are similar, pregabalin is absorbed more rapidly than gabapentin and pregabalin is absorbed proportional to the dose, whereas gabapentin exhibits absorption saturation so that the blood concentration does not increase proportionally to the dose. Although initially introduced as antiepileptic drugs, the gabapentinoids were not very effective in early clinical trials and would likely have been abandoned if not for studies showing that pregabalin was effective for treating chronic nerve pain associated with post-herpetic neuralgia (shingles) [21]. Subsequent studies showed modest benefit in patients with a variety of chronic pain syndromes, including fibromyalgia, and in patients with generalized anxiety and somatic symptoms. Only pregabalin is FDA-approved for treating neuropathic pain, but the gabapentinoids are the most widely prescribed drugs for off-label use in the United States today. Drug companies heavily marketed gabapentinoids for a variety of off-label uses particularly for treating anxiety and pain syndromes [22]. As with opioids, gabapentinoid abuse has become a major problem in the United States, with about 1.5% of people abusing gabapentinoids; many of these people were started on opioids and gabapentinoids for treating chronic back pain, despite the lack of evidence that either class of drugs is effective for treating chronic back pain. The most common side effects of the gabapentinoids are sedation, lethargy and dizziness, although these symptoms tend to diminish as patients develop tolerance to the medication. Gabapentinoids are sometimes used as sleeping pills, particularly in patients with chronic pain.

Anxiolytic Drugs

Drugs that enhance the inhibitory transmitter GABA, so-called GABA agonists, decrease excitatory transmission and are used for a variety of psychosomatic symptoms, particularly those associated with anxiety. Barbiturates, derived from barbituric acid, were the first class of GABA agonists. Bayer introduced phenobarbital (Luminal) in 1912 as a seizure drug, but by the mid-twentieth century barbiturates were being used for a broad range of psychosomatic symptoms. Addictions and deaths due to overdose became a major problem. By the latter twentieth century, barbiturates were largely replaced by a newer class of GABA agonists, benzodiazapines, which are anxiolytic but with much less overdose risk. Currently, benzodiazapines, diazepam (Valium), alprazolam (Xanax), lorazapam (Ativan) and clonazepam (Klonopin) are by far the most commonly prescribed drugs for anxiety in the United State and Europe [23]. But these drugs are not without risk. The decrease in excitatory transmission can result in sedation, fatigue, dizziness, prolonged reaction time, impaired driving skills and even impaired memory and cognitive function in older people. There is also a potential problem with tolerance (resulting in a patient's constant desire to increase the dose) and dependency (withdraw symptoms when stopping the drug) [24]. Unlike antidepressant drugs used for treating anxiety, benzodiazapines act rapidly and are not associated with initial jitteriness and insomnia. Sometimes benzdiazapines are used during the first few weeks of treatment with antidepressants to provide relief of anxiety until the antidepressant medications begin to have effect. As a rule, benzodiazapines are not useful for treating depression. Rapid- and short-acting lorazapam can be useful for treating panic attacks, preventing repeated emergency room visits.

Drugs that Enhance Neuroplasticity and Neurogenesis

As described in Chap. 5, a hallmark feature of chronic depression is shrinkage of the hippocampus with decreased neuroplasticity and neurogenesis. The nerve growth factor BDNF was shown to be an important mediator of neuroplasticity and neurogenesis, so drugs that enhanced BDNF activity were good candidate drugs for treating depression [25]. Injecting BDNF directly into the hippocampus of animals rapidly reversed depression induced by stress. Similar animal studies using the selective serotonin reuptake inhibitor fluoxetine found increased BDNF signaling and improved new synapse formation and neurogenesis, correlating with improved clinical symptoms, but a key limiting feature of fluoxetine and related antidepressant drugs is the long duration of weeks to months before clinical benefit occurs. During this critical delay period, suicides are disturbingly frequent. A more rapidly acting antidepressant medication was greatly needed. In 2000, clinical researchers reported that a short-acting anesthetic agent, ketamine, provided rapid antidepressant effects when given intravenously to patients with severe depression who failed other common treatments [26]. One such woman described the dramatic effects of intravenous ketamine. "After the first treatment, I felt a weight lift off me within hours. After three to four treatments, I could hear birds chirping and see vibrant colors again; I could walk out of the house without making a million excuses for why I couldn't. I had hope again. It was the first time in 20 years that I'd felt relief. And the results just kept getting better and better with each treatment" [27]. Subsequently, numerous clinical trials have documented the rapid effect of intravenous ketamine for treating major depression and an intranasal abbreviated form of ketamine has been developed and FDA-approved for treating depression.

Ketamine, The New "Wonder Drug"

Ketamine was developed at the pharmaceutical company Parke-Davis in the early 1960s as a short-acting anesthetic agent, and initial reports suggested relatively few side effects [17]. Although ketamine was used as a short-acting anesthetic agent for minor surgical procedures throughout the 1970s, particularly during the Vietnam War, bothersome side effects on wearing off became evident, including hallucinations, blood pressure spikes and muscle tremors. As newer, safer short-term anesthetics were developed, ketamine was largely abandoned for human surgical procedures, although it remains commonly used in veterinary medicine. In the 1990s ketamine became popular as a hallucinogenic recreational drug, often called "Special K." Users described visual and sound distortions, changes in body image and feelings of being disconnected from the body and reality, called the "K-hole." The duration of the effect was 30–60 min, much shorter than that of other recreational hallucinogenic drugs such as phencyclidine.

Ketamine acts on a variety of neurotransmitter systems, including monoamine and GABA receptors, but its most potent action is on the NMDA receptor of the excitatory transmitter glutamate, which in turn leads to increased BDNF production and release [28]. In rodent models of depression, ketamine rapidly increases synaptic protein production and reverses the stress-induced loss of synapses in the hippocampus and prefrontal cortex, correlating with rapid behavior response associated with improvement in depression. These changes are blocked in animals that are genetically engineered so that they can't produce BDNF. Ketamine also increases neurogenesis in the hippocampus in rodent models, but this takes days and probably accounts for the finding that a single dose of ketamine produces a sustained response for up to 7 days. Although intravenous ketamine has had a major impact on the treatment of severe depression, it is not an ideal drug considering the significant potential side effects and the inconvenience of having an intravenous infusion on a regular basis. Often benzodiazapines are used in combination with ketamine to ameliorate the psychoactive side effects. Drug companies immediately began searching for alternatives and developed a shortened version of ketamine, (S)-ketamine, that binds the NMDA receptor more tightly than regular ketamine and can be absorbed into the blood from a nasal spray. (S)-ketamine (Spravato) was approved by the FDA in 2020, and early studies suggest that it is highly effective for treating drug-resistant depression, but there are still no long term-trials regarding potentially serious side effects. The potential for abuse is also a major concern. Other drugs that bind the NMDA receptor but with fewer side effects than ketamine are being studied in both animal models and patients with depression, but so far the results have not been encouraging.

Remarkably, around the same time that ketamine was being evaluated for treating depression there were numerous reports of successful treatment with intravenous ketamine of severe chronic pain unresponsive to any other medications [29]. In one study, patients with refractory pain were anesthetized and maintained in a coma with ketamine for 5 days and when they awoke several had a dramatic relief of pain. Other studies using lower non-anesthetic intravenous doses found ketamine effective for treating a range of refractory chronic pain syndromes, including neuropathic pain, phantom limb pain, causalgia (currently called chronic regional pain syndrome) and fibromyalgia. But as with treating depression, side effects were a problem, and most studies were not adequately controlled for placebo effect. Despite the lack of evidence-based clinical trials, ketamine has become the "new wonder drug" for treating fibromyalgia/chronic fatigue syndrome, and many patients are paying thousands of dollars a month out of their own pocket for the treatment. Although initial reports are encouraging, we have a long way to go before understanding the role of ketamine and related drugs for treating depression and pain.

Drugs that Affect Endocannibinoid Neurotransmission

Although as noted in Chap. 5, the discovery of the endocannabinoid system and its role in the response to stress is relatively new, drugs that activate endocannabinoid receptors in the brain are some of the oldest drugs known to mankind. Ancient physicians in Asia and the Middle East used cannabis (marijuana) to treat pain, anxiety and depression several thousand years B.C. Cannabis was introduced to Western medicine in the mid-nineteenth century when the Irish born physician William O'Shaughnessy reported on his experience as an assistant surgeon in the East India Company traveling throughout India and the Middle East collecting information about the use of cannabis by local physicians. When he returned to England, his findings produced great excitement that rapidly spread to Europe and America. Despite this enthusiasm in the nineteenth century, the active ingredients in the marijuana plant and the brain cannabinoid receptors were not discovered until well into the twentieth century. Even with this new understanding, the role of cannabis and its derivatives as a medical treatment is still evolving and remains highly controversial.

Two main cannabinoid receptors, CB1 and CB2, have been identified in the brain [30]. Of the two, CB1 is most important for modulating the response to stress and anxiety. The CB1 effect on anxiety is highly dose-dependent such that low to moderate doses of cannabis relieve anxiety, whereas higher doses can cause or aggravate anxiety. Similarly, synthetic drugs with very high affinity for the CB1 receptor (so-called "spice" blends) are more likely to cause anxiety, panic and paranoid ideations. Many regular users of cannabis report that low to moderate doses produce relaxation, heightened sociability and creativity and even euphoria, whereas higher doses produce agitation, panic, cognitive impairment and rarely psychotic manifestations. But the cut-off between moderate and high-dose effect varies greatly among users, no doubt owing to a combination of genetic, developmental and contextual variables. The bidirectional action at the CB1 receptor results from its modulatory role in the release of glutamate and GABA in the amygdala and other limbic structures. These two main excitatory and inhibitory neurotransmitters affect anxiety in opposite directions so that low and high doses of drug may tip the balance between excitation and inhibition in either direction. In addition, the CB1 receptor has been shown to regulate the release of the monoamine neurotransmitters serotonin and noradrenalin and the hypothalamic-pituitary-adrenal axis and the release of stress hormones.

Cannabis was found to have two main active components, THC and CBD, each with opposite actions on the CB1 receptor [31]. THC is an agonist and CBD an antagonist. This in part explains why cannabis has a different overall effect than when either component is used alone. Both THC and CBD have actions on multiple neurotransmitter systems, so the end effect may not be predicted simply on the basis of the CB1 effect. Traditional marijuana plants contain about 20% THC and 1% CBD, although newer variants have higher CBD content [32]. There is a general consensus among marijuana users that THC will make you high while CBD will make you mellow, but this is an oversimplification (for reasons mentioned earlier). A wide variety of vaping oil, salve, tincture and edible products are made with predominant CBD, as high as 18/1, CBD/THC. Users report that these products produce anxiolytic effects without producing the typical marijuana high. In rodent models of anxiety, CBD reduces the amygdala response to fear and panic, an effect mediated through a serotonin receptor rather than the CB1 receptor. The ability of CBD and other cannabinoids to modulate animal emotional responses makes them attractive candidates for developing new drugs for treating anxiety, but the complexity of the cannabinoid role in regulating emotions and the potential for off-target effects and misuse liability have dampened the enthusiasm. For example, a cannabinoid mouth spray, Sativex, with a THC/CBD ration near 1/1, was marketed in Canada for treating chronic neuropathic pain, and although it is reasonably effective for controlling pain, it is not been effective for treating anxiety [33].

Of even greater concern are potential harmful effects of long-term use of cannabinoids [34, 35]. Emotional responses are often different in long-term versus occasional users of cannabis. Prolonged consumption can lead to lack of emotional awareness and motivation. Long-term administration of cannabinoids causes downregulation of the CB1 receptor, which may account for the altered emotional responses and may even lead to worsening of anxiety and other affective disorders. Studies in adolescents consistently found that chronic cannabis consumption leads to an increased risk for developing psychotic disorders, including schizophrenia

[36]. Furthermore, slight genetic variations in a gene that codes for an enzyme that degrades monoamines and psychosocial factors determine the magnitude of the risk. The complex interaction between nature and nurture in the production of psychogenic symptoms must be kept in mind when evaluating the effectiveness of new drugs.

Extracranial Brain Stimulation

Electroconvulsive Therapy (ECT)

As with many of the drugs used to treat psychogenic symptoms, ECT was discovered by accident when doctors observed that mentally ill patients who suffered from epilepsy often improved after having a seizure. Italian neurologist Ugo Cerletti performed the initial ECT treatments on patients in the 1930s [37]. According to psychiatric lore, Cerletti got the idea for ECT when he was shopping in a butcher shop and observed the butcher using electric shocks to the head of pigs to anesthetize them prior to being slaughtered. Cerletti experimented on inducing seizures in dogs by delivering electrical shocks to the head and then moved on to humans, reporting good results with ECT for a range of mental illnesses. By the 1940s, ECT was the new "wonder treatment" for severe mental illnesses at psychiatric hospitals around the world, and Cerletti was nominated for the Nobel Prize in Medicine. The scene of patients, strapped to tables with bite boards in their mouths, violently thrashing about and sometimes fracturing bones while in an induced seizure, was disturbing to many lay and medical professionals but the immediate benefit, particularly with severe depression, could not be denied. After a period of backlash against what many considered an inhumane treatment in the 1960s and 1970s, ECT made a comeback in part due to the use of general anesthesia to prevent the convulsive movements. Even in the twenty-first century, it is widely used around the world with an estimated one million ECT treatments performed yearly [38].

How does ECT work? Some have likened it to rebooting a computer, but this is an obvious oversimplification. After the procedure, patients do not remember the event or events around the time of the procedure. With initial treatments, memory typically recovers over weeks but in some, particularly with those with repeated treatments, memory loss is permanent. People also report difficulties with concentration and attention and even confusion after the procedure, and as with memory loss these symptoms are more common and persistent in people who have received numerous treatment courses. ECT produces a burst of excitatory neurotransmission in the brain followed by a rebound of inhibitory neurotransmission [39]. A pulsed release of monoamine neurotransmitters activates neuroplasticity and neurogenesis in the hippocampus much more rapidly than with antidepressant drugs. Although ECT has primarily been used for treating severe depression, recent studies suggest it might also be useful for treating chronic pain including fibromyalgia/chronic fatigue syndrome [40]. ECT appears to decrease central sensitization to pain and improve blood flow to key pain centers. But what price is being paid for the short-term benefits of ECT on overall brain health? As a neurologist who has seen many patients with poorly controlled generalized epileptic seizures slowly lose cognitive abilities, it is common sense to be concerned about the practice of inducing repeat seizures to treat poorly understood psychogenic illnesses. Fortunately, preliminary studies suggest that intravenous ketamine may be as effective for treating severe depression as ECT, so there may be a less dangerous option for dealing with these terrible illnesses until more effective targeted treatments are developed [41].

Transcranial Direct Current Stimulation (tDCS)

A less risky method for presenting focused electrical stimulation of the brain, tDCS has been around since the 1960s. It was initially used by neurologists to help with recovery after stroke. More recently tDCS has been applied to a variety of psychogenic illness, including depression, anxiety, PTSD and fibromyalgia/chronic fatigue syndrome with the goal of improving neuroplasticity. The procedure is well tolerated with few side effects. With tDCS, a weak direct electrical current of 1–2 mA is applied directly to the scalp through paste-on electrodes on each side of the head, usually in the prefrontal region. Changes in cortical excitability last for hours after stimulation, and the increase in excitatory neurotransmission presumably enhances long-term potentiation at neuronal synapses. Initial clinical trials suggest tDCS may be helpful as a primary or adjuvant treatment for depression and PTSD, but better-controlled treatment trials are needed before its beneficial effects are proven [42, 43].

Transcranial Magnetic Stimulation (TMS)

The latest panacea for treating psychogenic illnesses is TMS [44]. Unlike ECT and tDCS, which use electrical current to stimulate nerves and neurons, TMS uses a magnetic field generator (coil) that delivers magnetic impulses to activate regions of the brain under the coil. The magnitude of the magnetic field is about 1.5 Tesla, which is similar to the magnetic field in an MRI machine, although with TMS the magnetic field is on for brief pulses compared to the constant field with an MRI machine. Side effects appear to be minimal with the most common being headache. The internet is filled with advertisements for TMS for treating depression, tinnitus (ringing in the ears), chronic dizziness, chronic pain, post-traumatic stress disorder (PTSD) and fibromyalgia/chronic fatigue syndrome. The procedure is only FDA-approved for treating depression, and controlled treatment trials for depression show a modest 30–50% response rate after a course of treatment, usually with the coil over the prefrontal cortex. This region of the brain was chosen because the prefrontal cortex is known to be involved in depression and it is the easiest brain region to access with the coil. A typical treatment course is 5 days a week for 4–6 weeks, and desperate patients are paying large amounts of money out of pocket because insurance companies usually will not pay for the procedure. Currently, there are not enough high-quality treatment trials to prove efficacy with TMS, even for treating depression [45]. One must keep in mind that the placebo response rate in drug trials for most psychogenic illnesses, including depression, is in the range of 30–50%, and complex technological treatments like TMS and tDCS with elaborate rituals probably have an even higher placebo effect rate.

Deep Brain Stimulation

An obvious problem with treating psychogenic illnesses using external brain stimulation is the lack of focus of the stimulation. Large areas of the brain are activated, parts of which may be important in generating symptoms while other parts may have nothing to do with the symptoms or even may be suppressing symptoms. A possible solution to this problem is to implant tiny electrodes in the brain in critical centers known to be involved in generating the symptoms, so-called deep brain stimulation (DBS). Although relatively safe, a surgical procedure is required to insert the electrodes, so all of the routine risks of surgery apply. One must also keep in mind that even tiny electrodes activate large numbers of neurons and nerve fibers passing through that may in turn activate distant neurons. Key questions yet to be answered are which areas should be stimulated and what type of stimuli should be used? Depending on the stimulus parameters, an electrode can excite or inhibit neurons and nerve fiber tracks in the region. For example, high-frequency (>100 Hz) stimulation can inactivate nerve cell bodies but activate nerve fibers passing by. DBS can also trigger release of neurotransmitters and induce neuroplasticity. We are currently in the wild, wild west regarding evaluating the risk/benefits of intracranial stimulation for psychogenic symptoms. Some even question whether it is ethical to consider a treatment that can potentially alter a person's feelings and personality.

Early studies using open-loop DBS for treating obsessive-compulsive disorder (OCD), depression and post-traumatic stress disorder (PTSD) have produced mixed results. Open-loop means that the stimulus parameters for the electrode are pre-programmed at the time of insertion and then adjusted at follow-up visits (usually monthly) based on the patient's subjective report of benefits and side effects. Although initial uncontrolled clinical trials of DBS for major depression were encouraging, two randomized controlled treatment trials were terminated early owing to negative results [46]. Numerous potential problems could explain the negative results, including choosing the wrong location for the electrodes, slight misplacement of the electrodes, difficulties programming the electrodes based on the patient's subjective reports and the lack of any objective measure that the target circuits are being stimulated. At the present time, the only DBS treatment available outside of research protocols in the United States is open-loop DBS for treating patients with OCD, which has a Humanitarian Devise Exemption from the FDA [47].

DBS for PTSD

There has been a great deal of interest in the use of DBS for treating PTSD, probably because of the large number of people with this debilitating illness and the lack of effective treatments [48]. A brief review of the theoretical underpinning and preliminary clinical trials of DBS for PTSD provides a good glimpse of where we are currently and where the future may be for DBS treatment of psychogenic illnesses. As discussed in Chap. 5, the amygdala, hippocampus and prefrontal cortex are key parts of a fear/anxiety network. In animal models, the basolateral region of the amygdala (BLA) appears to be important for fear memories and persistent fear responses. The prefrontal cortex normally controls the BLA modulating fear responses, and a simple working hypothesis to explain PTSD is that loss of prefrontal inhibition of the BLA causes fear memories to dominate emotional responses [49]. Studies in a rodent model of PTSD show that stimulation of an electrode implanted in the BLA improves fear conditioning and fear-related behaviors, and recently electrodes were implanted into the BLA of a few veterans suffering from refractory PTSD [42]. Although preliminary results with open-loop devises in the BLA are encouraging, there are problems with programing and measuring effectiveness of the devises. Without a biological marker for symptom severity, the stimulation parameters are set based on periodic reports from the patient, which are highly subjective and constantly changing. By nature, PTSD is an episodic disorder, so that continuous stimulation during periods when the patient is not having symptoms may be inappropriate. Most investigators feel that the future of DBS is with some form of closed-loop stimulation. Closed-loop means that biological markers such as activation of the autonomic nervous system, stress hormone levels in the blood or neuronal activity in another brain region provide the signal that determines the firing pattern of the stimulating electrode. For example, decreases in electrodermal conduction associated with sweating or increases in heart rate and blood pressure could be a biological marker for stress and used to control the firing pattern in the amygdala to alleviate the stress related symptoms. Interestingly, a smart phone app has been developed using a similar strategy, whereby the user wears an instrument that monitors autonomic nervous system responses and communicates with the smartphone to deliver soothing, relaxing messages to the wearer when the measurements indicate stress and anxiety [50]. The ultimate and potentially most controversial closed-loop DBS is to use activity in one part of the brain to control the activity in another part of the brain. In the case of PTSD, a logical closed-loop system might be to monitor activity in the prefrontal cortex to control stimulation in the BLA. With recent advances in microelectrode technology, it is possible to record and stimulate from hundreds of microelectrodes in both locations so that one could fine tune the connections between the prefrontal cortex and BLA electrodes. Even with these multi-electrode arrays, however, the communication between brain centers will still be crude compared to the normal-functioning brain, and unintended side effects of the chronic stimulation are of concern.

In Brief

People with psychosomatic symptoms do best within a structured lifestyle that includes regular physical exercise, adequate time for sleep, healthy eating habits and stress management techniques such as mindfulness, yoga and tai chi.

Cognitive-behavioral therapy can help patients recognize and modify thoughts and activities that trigger symptoms. Numerous drugs, including antidepressants, anti-epileptics and anxiolytics, are used to treat psychosomatic symptoms, but none have been dramatically effective. A major limitation of these drugs is "off-target effects" that lead to bothersome side effects and variable response. Transcranial direct current stimulation (tDCS) and transcranial magnetic stimulation (TMS) are promising new treatments for a variety of psychosomatic illnesses, but well-controlled treatment trials are needed to access efficacy and safety.

Future Directions

It is common sense that medical professionals must become more committed to prescribing exercise for their patients and regularly checking on compliance, just as they do with any other prescription. Patients need to understand how important exercise is for brain health and how effective it is for a wide variety of psychogenic illnesses, in many cases better than any drug currently available. A discussion of lifestyle and its effect on psychogenic symptoms should be a part of any treatment plan. Such a plan might consist of a regular exercise routine, daily mindfulness sessions, and cognitive behavioral therapy. These conditions tend to be chronic, so patients need to develop a long-term strategy for living with them. The news and social media already influence people's perception of psychogenic illness, and this will only increase in the future. Numerous apps are available for monitoring exercise and for teaching relaxation techniques, including mindfulness. On-line psychotherapy is in the early stages but has the potential to reach large segments of the public who would otherwise not have access to such therapy. Long-term effectiveness of on-line treatments and how this should be evaluated needs to be worked out. On the other hand, reading and ruminating about news stories and people's blogs describing their symptoms can worsen symptoms in people who are already fearful and worrying about their symptoms. There is a delicate balance between being informed and information overload.

A major limitation for treating psychosomatic symptoms with drugs is their lack of specificity. Drugs that target a specific protein have effects everywhere in the brain that the protein is expressed, not just the neural connections producing the symptoms. Furthermore, drugs have multiple targets; even drugs that have high affinity for a particular neurotransmitter or receptor have off-target effects. With improved understanding of the nerve pathways involved in specific psychogenic illnesses, it will be possible to develop more potent drugs for suppressing symptoms, but there will always be unexpected side effects. As susceptibility variants in genes for different psychogenic illnesses become better understood, it will be necessary to obtain an individual's genetic profile to minimize side effects of any new drug. Two areas where future drug treatments show the most promise are for chronic pain and depression. The underlying brain abnormalities for these disorders are reasonably well understood, and the symptoms are so incapacitating that patients are more willing to accept side effects as long as the pain and depression improve. It may be possible to identify drug targets that are relatively specific to the disorders with minimal off-target effects. For example, certain target proteins, such as ion channels, are highly specific for pain pathways with little expression elsewhere, so that targeting these proteins can suppress pain but have little effect on non-pain brain pathways. Of course, off-target effects are always possible and may only show up when the drugs are tested in large clinical trials.

Although brain stimulation either externally or internally has exciting potential for treating a small subset of people with psychogenic illness, obvious limitations include lack of localization with external stimulation and risks of surgery with internal stimulation. Furthermore, long-term adverse effects with either type of stimulation have not been adequately evaluated. One can only hope that ECT will become a historical footnote as better treatments, such as intravenous ketamine, are developed for severe depression. TMS has relatively few known side effects and is well tolerated but exactly what is being achieved with the stimulation is unclear, and further evaluation in animal models of depression and chronic pain is required. Widespread use of the technique simply because it is relatively safe, before there is better understanding of the short- and long-term effects, makes no sense. At the least, large, randomized, placebo (sham stimulation) controlled treatment trials are needed to document efficacy. Finally, although DBS has the potential for dramatic results in patients with intractable severe depression and chronic pain, we are still a long way from understanding the best locations and stimulation techniques. There appears to be a consensus that closed-loop stimulation is the future for DBS, but what measurements are used for feedback to the stimulating electrodes is yet to be determined. The most promising technique is to use activity in one region of the brain to control the firing of electrodes in another region of the brain. But the long-term consequences and the ethics of placing electrodes in key emotional centers of the brain require future investigation and political discourse.

References

1. Conrad P. The shifting engines of medicalization. J Health Soc Behav. 2005;46:11.
2. Herring BP, Puetz TW, O'Conner PJ, Dishman RK. Effect of exercise training on depressive symptoms and meta-analysis of randomized controlled trials. Arch Intern Med. 2012;172:101–11.
3. Stonerock GL, Hoffman BM, Smith PJ, Blumenthal JA. Exercise as treatment for anxiety: systematic review and analysis. Ann Behav Med. 2015;49:542–56.
4. Roeh A, Kirchner SK, Malchow B, et al. Depression in somatic disorders: is there a beneficial effect of exercise. Front Psych. 2019;10:141.
5. Chekroud SR, Gueorguieva R, Zheutlin AB, et al. Association between physical exercise and mental health in 1.2 million individuals in the USA between 2011 and 2015: a cross-sectional study. Lancet Psychiatry. 2018;5:739–46.
6. Xu Z, Hu M, Wang Z, et al. The positive effect of moderate-intensity exercise on the mirror neuron system: an fNIRS study. Front Psychol. 2019;10:986.
7. James W. The principles of psychology. New York: Holt; 1890.
8. Gu J, Strauss C, Bond R, Cavanagh K. How do mindfulness-based cognitive therapy and mindfulness-based stress reduction improve mental health and wellbeing? A systematic review and meta-analysis of meditation studies. Clin Psychol Rev. 2015;37:1–12.

9. Hofmann SG, Gomez AF. Mindfulness-based interventions for anxiety and depression. Psychiatr Clin North Am. 2017;40:739–49.
10. Brewin C. Theoretical foundations of cognitive-behavioral therapy for anxiety and depression. Ann Rev Psychol. 1996;47:33–57.
11. Baardseth TP, Goldberg SB, Pace BT, et al. Cognitive-behavioral therapy versus other therapies: Redux. Clin Psychol Rev. 2013;33:395–405.
12. Hofmann SG, Asmundson GJG. Acceptance and mindfulness-based therapy: new wave or old hat? Clin Psychol Rev. 2008;28:1–16.
13. Andersson G, Titov N, Dear BF, et al. Internet-delivered psychological treatments: from innovation to implementation. World Psychiatry. 2019;18:20–8.
14. Arnberg FK, Linton SJ, Hultcrantz M, et al. Internet-delivered psychological treatments for mood and anxiety disorders: a systematic review of their efficacy, safety, and cost-effectiveness. PLoS One. 2019;9:e98118.
15. Kelson J, Rollin A, Ridout B, Campbell A. Internet-delivered acceptance and commitment therapy for anxiety treatment: systematic review. J Med Internet Res. 2019;21:e12530.
16. Hirschfeld RMA. History and evolution of the monoamine hypothesis depression. J Clin Psychiatry. 2000;61(Suppl 6):4–6.
17. Hillhouse TM, Porter JH. A brief history of the development of antidepressant drugs: from monoamine to glutamate. Exp Clin Psychopharmacol. 2015;23:1–21.
18. Shaw DM, Eccleston EG, Camps FE. 5-Hydroxytriptamine in the hind-brain of depressive suicides. Br J Psychiatry. 1967;113:1407–11.
19. Wong DT, Perry KW, Bymaster FP. The discovery of fluoxetine hydrochloride (Prozac). Nat Rev Drug Discov. 2005;4:764–74.
20. Stahl SM, Grady MM, Moret C, Briley M. SNRIs: their pharmacology, clinical efficacy, and tolerability in comparison with other classes of antidepressants. CNS Spectr. 2005;10:732–47.
21. Dworkin RH, Corbin AE, Young JP Jr, et al. Pregabalin for the treatment of postherpetic neuralgia: a randomized, placebo-controlled trial. Neurology. 2003;60:1274–83.
22. Lauria-Horner BA, Pohl RB. Pregabalin: a new anxiolytic. Expert Opin Investig Drugs. 2003;12:663–72.
23. Stahl SM. Don't ask, don't tell, but benzodiazepines are still the leading treatments for anxiety disorder. J Clin Psychiatry. 2002;63(9):756–7.
24. Livingston MG. Benzodiazepine dependence. Br J Hosp Med. 1994;51(6):281–6.
25. Notaras M, van den Buuse M. Brain –derived neurotrophic factor (BDNF): novel insights into regulation and genetic variation. Neuroscientist. 2019;25:434–54.
26. Berman RM, Cappiello A, Anand A, et al. Antidepressant effects of ketamine in depressed patients. Biol Psychiatry. 2000;47:351–4.
27. Johnson C. A ketamine revolution for depression and pain? Spravato, fibromyalgia and ME/CFS. www.healthrising. Blog, 2019/04/20.
28. Deyama S, Duman R. Neurotrophic mechanisms underlying the rapid and sustained antidepressant action of ketamine. Pharmacol Biochem Behav. 2020;188:1–9.
29. Niesters M, Martini C, Dahan A. Ketamine for chronic pain: risks and benefits. Br J Clin Pharmacol. 2013;77:357–67.
30. Tambaro S, Bortolato M. Cannabinoid-related agents in the treatment of anxiety disorders: current knowledge and future perspectives. Recent Pat CNS Drug Discov. 2012;7:25–40.
31. Bhattacharyya S, Morrison PD, Fusar-Poli P, et al. Opposite effects of delta-9-tetrahydrocannabinol and cannabidiol on human brain function and psychopathology. Neuropsychopharmacology. 2010;35(3):764–74.
32. ElSohly MA, Slade D. Chemical constituents of marijuana: the complex mixture of natural cannabinoids. Life Sci. 2005;78:539–48.
33. Karschner EL, Darwin WD, McMahon RP, et al. Subjective and physiological effects after controlled Sativex and oral THC administration. Clin Pharmacol Ther. 2011;89:400–7.
34. Millman RB, Sbriglio R. Patterns of use and psychopathology in chronic marijuana users. Psychiatr Clin North Am. 1986;9:533–45.
35. Hall W, Solowij N. Adverse effects of cannabis. Lancet. 1998;352:1611–6.

36. Murray RM, Morrison PD, Henquet C, Di Forti M. Cannabis, the mind and society: the harsh realities. Nat Rev Neurosci. 2007;8:885–95.
37. Lieberman JA, Ogas O. Shrinks: the untold story of psychiatry. New York: Little, Brown; 2015.
38. Leiknes KA, Jarosh-von Schweder L, Høie B. Contemporary use and practice of electroconvulsive therapy worldwide. Brain Behav. 2012;2:283–344.
39. Newman ME, Gur E, Shapira B, Lerer B. Neurochemical mechanisms of action of ECS: evidence from in vivo studies. J ECT. 1998;14:153–71.
40. Usui C, Doi N, Nishioka M, et al. Electroconvulsive therapy improves severe pain associated with fibromyalgia. Pain. 2006;121:276–80.
41. Kheirabadi G, Vafaie M, Kheirabadi D, et al. Comparative effect of intravenous ketamine and electroconvulsive therapy in major depression: a randomized controlled trial. Adv Biomed Res. 2019;8:25.
42. Gouveia FV, Gidyk DC, Giacobbe P, et al. Neuromodulation strategies in post-traumatic stress disorder: from preclinical models to clinical applications. Brain Sci. 2019;9:45.
43. Bennabi D, Haffen E. Transcranial direct current stimulation (tDCS): a promising treatment for major depressive disorder. Brain Sci. 2018;8:81.
44. Perera T, George MS, Grammer G, et al. The clinical TMS Society consensus review and treatment recommendations for TMS therapy for major depressive disorder. Brain Stimul. 2016;9:336–46.
45. Couturier JL. Efficacy of rapid-rate repetitive transcranial magneticstimulation in the treatment of depression: a systematic review and meta-analysis. J Psychiatry Neurosci. 2005;30(2):83–90.
46. Lo M-C, Widge AS. Closed-loop neuromodulation systems: next-generation treatments for psychiatric illness. Int Rev Psychiatry. 2017;29:191–204.
47. Greenberg BD, Gabriels LA, Malone DA, et al. Deep brain stimulation of the ventral internal capsule/ventral striatum for obsessive-compulsive disorder: worldwide experience. Mol Psychiatry. 2010;15:64–79.
48. Lavano A, Guzzy G, Della Torre A, et al. DBS in treatment of post-traumatic stress disorder. Brain Sci. 2018;8:18.
49. Bina RW, Langevin J-P. Closed loop brain stimulation for PTSD, addiction, and disorders of affective facial interpretation: review and discussion of potential biomarkers and stimulation paradigms. Front Neurosci. 2018;12:300.
50. Fletcher RR, Tam S, Omojola O, et al. Wearable sensor platform and mobile application for use in cognitive behavioral therapy for drug addiction and PTSD. Conf Proc IEEE Eng Med Biol Soc. 2011;2011:1802–5.

Index